YOU HAVE to PUT GOLD

into the FIRE

to PURIFY IT.

Yoga the Sacred Science
volume three

SAMYAMA
The Power of Self-Transformation

**Yoga the Sacred Science
volume three**

Swami Rama

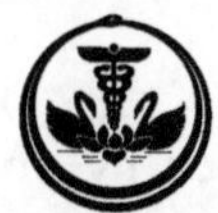

Himalayan Institute Hospital Trust
Swami Rama Nagar, P.O. Jolly Grant
Dehradun - 248016, Uttarakhand, India

Acknowledgements

We would like to express our appreciation to Connie Gage for designing the cover and to Wesley Van Linda for his assistance in publishing this book. A special thanks to Kamal for book production. Also, again thanks to Swami Jnaneshwara for sharing his version of bhuta shuddhi. And finally, we are grateful to Turiya and Sandhya for their loving assistance with the Sanskrit terms.

Editing: Dr. Barbara Bova
Cover design: Connie Gage

©2024 Himalayan Institute Hospital Trust

ISBN 978-81-956296-8-8

Published by:
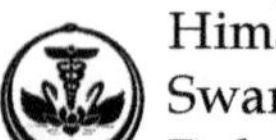 Himalayan Institute Hospital Trust
Swami Rama Nagar, P.O. Jolly Grant
Dehradun - 248016, Uttarakhand, India
Tel: 91-135-247-1233, Fax: 91-135-247-1141
src@hihtindia.org; www.hihtindia.org

Distributed by Lotus Press, P.O. Box 325, Twin Lakes, WI 53181 U.S.A., www.lotuspress.com, 800-824-6396, lotuspress@lotuspress.com

Table of Contents

Foreword

Samyama, the Power of Self-Transformation is Volume 3 of *Yoga the Sacred Science*, Swami Rama's comments on Patanjali's Yoga Sutras and the science of yoga in general. This volume completes the series. Volumes 1 *(Samadhi)* and 2 *(Sadhana)* describe the systematic practice of the science of yoga, with a focus on the healing of psyche and soma through gaining control of mind and its modifications and practising the basics of holistic health according to Ashtanga Yoga. Volume 3 *(Samyama)* describes the final steps of Ashtanga Yoga that lead to self-healing, self-transformation and samadhi, or enlightenment, and the consequent acquisition of siddhis (powers). I have chosen to present the general topic of samyama in the early part of the book and have included the powers that are attained from the practice of samyama later under the topic *Siddhis*.

Although Patanjali does not specifically mention kundalini and techniques for awakening the kundalini, Swami Rama was a yoga master, who went through a highly disciplined training far beyond anything we could imagine in all aspects and philosophies of yoga. In his lectures and writings he often mixes the different philosophies, making it difficult to siphon out only Patanjali's Yoga. For this reason I have included kundalini and tantra as necessary addendums to the discussion of Patanjali's Sutras and the process of self-transformation.

Swamiji spent all the years he was with us teaching the essence of Patanjali's Yoga Sutras along with the undisputable wisdom of the ancient Vedas and the incomparable knowledge of the sacred Upanishads. He repeatedly stressed the importance of a healthy body and mind as necessary requisites to the practice of meditation. Those persons who came to learn yoga at Swamiji's Himalayan Institute in Pennsylvania were enrolled in the Self-Transformation Program (STP). This practical residential program included lectures, seminars, hatha yoga training, breath and relaxation training, dietary guidance and meditation, along with Karma Yoga, all according to the teachings of Patanjali, the Vedas and the Upanishads. And so, I have taken the liberty of creating an amalgam of all of Swamiji's diverse yet inseparable teachings in one cauldron of truth, rather than restricting the topics of this volume simply to Patanjali. I trust this will not only be acceptable to those persons who choose to embark on the sacred journey to self-transformation, but will also encourage them to use their inner strength to take their journey to its limitless unfathomable goal of the highest state of consciousness as pursued by the ancient sages. Many names are used to refer to the highest state of consciousness such as: center of consciousness, pure consciousness, Atman, Brahman, the Self, God, Allah, absolute reality, truth, the Lord, Bhagwan, Ishvara and Yahweh. Regardless of which religion they come from, they all refer to the one pure consciousness that is beyond all dualities, body, senses, conscious mind and unconscious mind, and that resides within every human being.

In 1976 I was blessed to have been one of the students in Swamiji's course on the Yoga Sutras, the first graduate level course taught at the Himalayan Institute of Glenview, IL. For me, that course marked the beginning of a lifetime study and practice of the science of yoga, which evolved to include the study and practice of homeopathic medicine. The basic goals common to both are self-healing, self-training and self-transformation. The word *transformation* evokes the ancient science of alchemy. The common Sanskrit term for alchemy is *rasaśāstra,* "the teaching on mercury."

Edward C. Whitmont, M.D. was a highly respected homeopath and Jungian psychoanalyst of the twentieth century. In his book, *The Alchemy of Healing,* he described the process of self-healing and self-transformation as similar to the alchemical transformation of a base metal into gold. In yoga, the alchemical transformation is of lower consciousness to the highest level of consciousness or samadhi. In homeopathy, the transformation that takes place activates self-healing not only of psyche and soma but also at the deepest spiritual level. Whitmont writes:

"The alchemists held that the transformation of base substances into gold constituted the bringing forth and purifying of an innermost divine essence that lies dormant in earthly existence. This process was considered tantamount to a "healing" of "diseased" substance. The *lapis philosophorum* (philosopher's stone) that was to catalyze this transformation could be created only through a process that involved both the substance to be worked upon and the operator's soul and personality. Transformation, purification and generation of the eternal Self on a psyche-substance level was a quasi-cosmic healing. Mundane healing, in turn, amounted to a psyche-substance transformation moving toward a transpersonal Self, toward an immanency that both prefigured and was the goal of existence.

"To the alchemist's holistic view, transformation and healing were equivalent. Through transmutation into gold, all substance is redeemed from the imperfections of its "incarnation" into form. This gold, however, is not to be confused with the ordinary gold, the *aurum vulgi,* but is the "essence" of "pure" implicate order expression, a symbolic manifestation of sun and spirit, brought about by human effort and divine grace. Failure to accomplish this was tantamount to illness, both of substance as well as of soul and body. Hence healing was to be prefigured to genuine transformation of body, soul and spirit.

"In the transformational context of the alchemical parameter and of homeopathy, healing aims at a restoration of individual integrity, vibrancy and at-oneness with the Self and with the world-totality, akin to the alchemist's idea of making or refining "gold.""[1]

In November 1992 Swamiji conducted a lecture series in a retreat at Mt. Kota Kinabalu, the highest mountain in Malaysia. On the second day of the retreat he did a number of demonstrations:

---

1 Whitmont, Edward C., M.D. *The Alchemy of Healing.* Berkely, California, North Atlantic Books, 1993. Pp. 47-49.

Swami Rama:

"The demonstrations I am about to do I have rarely done outside the lab previously. I want students to learn something so that they practise, so that this tradition remains alive. Otherwise it will die."

Then, he proceeded to rub mercury into the palm of his left hand, after which he immediately excreted the mercury in his urine. He had demonstrated the same in 1964 as described by a witness who was present at that time:

Around 1964, Swamiji was living in a small cottage built in a garden at Sitapur, a city about 50 miles from Lucknow, the capital of Utter Pradesh. One day Swamiji asked me to bring some pure mercury. I didn't know where to get pure mercury but finally purchased two thermometers, broke their mercury reservoirs and collected the mercury. Before giving it to Swamiji, I ensured there was no piece of glass in it. Then Swamiji put that mercury in the palm of his left hand, put a few drops of water on it and rubbed the mercury into his palm. After about three to four minutes, except for a visible grey mark in his palm, there was no mercury remaining in his palm. Thinking it might have spilled from his hand I searched for the mercury on the floor but couldn't see any. He pretended he did not know the whereabouts of the mercury and asked me where it had gone. Then, he said it probably had gone into his body. I became very worried, as mercury is poisonous. We kept talking for some time about this and the possible consequences. He then said there was no need to worry because he would pass out the total amount of mercury from his body through the urine. I provided him a glass tumbler and indeed he passed out all the mercury along with the urine into that tumbler.

Back at the retreat later that evening we asked Swamiji to explain how he was able to absorb the mercury into the body. He replied, "You have to be able to create a temperature of 150 degrees C and completely stop the flow of apana in order to absorb the mercury. If you have a liter of oil and you heat it until it vaporizes, you will have the same amount, a liter of oil vapor. There is a hollow tube in the body — the centralis canalis. I took the mercury into my blood and then into the centralis canalis to the brain. Because no one would know what I had done, I excreted it from the blood into the urine."

"Why would you take it to the brain?"

"Mercury is very powerful and can regenerate brain cells."

We continued our interrogation:

"Is that what alchemy really is?"

"Yes, the conversion of mercury to vapor."

"Is that the philosopher's stone?"

"Yes. The gold in alchemy is knowledge."

"Did Jung understand alchemy?"

"Yes. So did Socrates, Aristotle and Plato."

"Did Hahnemann (the founder of homeopathy)?"

"Yes."

"Does anyone else know?"

"There is one other person in my tradition that I taught. I started to play around with mercury when I was seven years old, but not until I was 19 did I start to use it without supervision. That is our tradition."

Then Swamiji told us another story about gold:

In my travels I met one swami who was able to make gold. I was very impressed with him and decided to become his disciple. I told my master good-bye, that I had found another guru who could teach me how to make gold. He said fine and asked me what his name was. I told him and asked him if he knew him. My master said at one time that person had been his student but had left the monastery. Then my master called me goldsmith and asked me to bring a rock. I left to find a rock and gave it to him when I returned, and he pissed on it. Before my eyes, half of it turned into gold! I thought maybe it was just the outside that was covered with gold so I broke a piece off and sold it. It was solid gold.

When we asked him if he still had that rock he replied that he did and that he also could make gold, but the cost was outrageous. In order to make a piece of gold worth $100, you would have to spend $100,000 (in energy)!

Remember, all that glitters is not gold.

Dr. Barbara Bova
Himalayan Institute Hospital Trust
Jolly Grant, Dehradun, India

INTRODUCTION

BRAHMAN
the MANIFESTATION
the POWER that MAKES a HUMAN BEING
THREE SELVES
the EVOLUTION of SPIRITUALITY
VEDAS
PATANJALI'S YOGA SUTRAS
YOGA SCIENCE and YOGA PSYCHOLOGY
SCIENCE of SELF-DEVELOPMENT

BRAHMAN

As described in *Mundaka Upanishad,* fire is the head and the moon and sun are the eyes of Brahman; all four directions are the ears. Brahman's speech encompasses all the knowledge contained in Vedic literature. Air is its prana and this universe is its heart; earth itself has emerged from its feet and it alone is the inner Self of all living beings.

The word *Brahman* is derived from the Sanskrit verb root *brh* meaning "expansion, knowledge or all-pervasiveness." This word is always of a neuter gender because it represents the absolute reality beyond the concept of male or female and all other dualities. Brahman is that which alone exists and allows the entire universe to appear within itself. Brahman is omnipresent, omniscient and omnipotent; it is the very nature of one's true Self. That absolute reality, that supreme pure consciousness, which is never affected by the ever-changing nature of the world, is Brahman. The entire universe is a manifestation of that pure consciousness. The waves of truth, beauty and wisdom are part of this great ocean of bliss. You may feel you are different from Brahman, but the scriptures say you are identical to Brahman. Brahman is no different from oneself; all of humanity is Brahman. From this point of view, all people are essentially one and the same. To place duality and diversity within humanity is the greatest loss; to realize the oneness within and without is the highest gain. Because of intoxication you see two where there is only one. The difference between hypnosis and meditation is this. Whereas diversity is the result of hypnosis, meditation will lead you to unity. Although we are many different faces within the principle of diversity, there is oneness beneath our apparent existence. If everyone were to withdraw from body consciousness and mind consciousness, it would be more obvious we are all one. If you were constantly aware of that oneness, you could never hurt, harm or injure anyone. Instead, everyone would be working for each other. You would be free because you would be doing your actions and giving the fruits of your actions to others, and they would be doing the same for you.

Those who are aware of that unity in diversity can easily get freedom. You identify with your thoughts and with things that are subject to change, death and decay, and that is why you are suffering. You have forgotten your true nature, which is peace, happiness and wisdom. I'm talking about your soul that dwells within you but is beyond body, breath, senses and mind. The moment you become aware of that, you will realize that happiness that cannot be robbed by your mind, thoughts, desires or emotions.

When I meditate, I do not see your many faces, but only that one unity, one life force that is beneath all these beautiful faces. Meditation helps you to know yourself on all levels. You have to simply go within to the center of silence where the absolute reality resides in all its glory. Once you know your Self, you will know the Self of all.

THE MANIFESTATION

When pure consciousness manifests itself, it divides into two aspects: the ultimate reality and the power of manifestation, which is the creative or dynamic principle. Therefore, all energy exists in two forms: latent and dynamic. Subsequently, all activities or forces of motion have a static background. In VEDANTA philosophy these two principles are referred to as Paramatman and Mahamaya. Thus, you all are sparks of Paramatman, bubbles in the great ocean of the universe. Atman is perfect and unalloyed and pervades both the internal and external worlds. Atman's nature is pure happiness and bliss. This jewel is deeply buried in the tomb of your body. Without destroying that tomb or hurting any part of yourself, you have to gently dig out that jewel.

In SAMKHYA and YOGA these two principles are referred to as Purusha and Prakriti. *Puru* means "city," *sha* means "sleeping." One who is sleeping in the city of life is called Purusha. Purusha is another name for Atman, your soul. According to Samkhya and yoga science, the essence of all is Purusha consciousness, the sleeping dormant power. Once you allow it to awaken and grow, you will be able to do wonders in the world. One who knows Purusha residing in the cave of the heart that is situated between the upper hemisphere and lower hemisphere, can destroy the knot of ignorance that creates bondage and gives many fears, depression, pains and misery. You can liberate yourself from that. That sleeping consciousness within you is a seed. If I have a seed in my hand and I tell you I am holding a tree, you might think something odd has happened to me. But actually, what I am saying is true. The seed contains a tree, and even flowers and fruits. You are just not seeing it. If I tell you I have fruits in my hand but all you see is a little seed, I am right and you are also right. I am right because if you allow this seed to grow, the seed will break and it will become a tree. There are two powers inside the seed that can throw roots downward into the ground and also grow upward. Then it gives flowers followed by fruits, so I am not wrong. The essence of the tree, flowers and fruits is in the seed. That seed contains everything.

One of the homeopathic doctors in Germany said someone told him, "What a foolish thing you have done. After doing MD and surgery, you have become a homeopath. How is it possible to cure someone by giving only a drop of medicine? This is stupid."

Then the homeopath replied, "You have forgotten that you also were made out of a drop. One drop is quite sufficient."

From Prakriti evolves prana, the life energy. Just as a man plants a seed in a woman and life ensues, so with the aid of Purusha do numberless beings evolve from Prakriti. There is a controversy about when life enters into the fertilized ovum. Life is already there but it is in unmanifested form. You cannot kill life in unmanifested form. Nothing happens to life; life goes to life. The moment the sperm is received by the ovum is the actual moment of birth, because life is already there. When you start to breathe, you become a human being. The ancients knew how to discipline themselves, so wife and husband used to meet only occasionally to bring a child into the world.

According to TANTRA philosophy, the inseparable male and female principles are called Shiva and Shakti. Shiva remains absorbed in the deepest state of meditation in a state of formless being, consciousness and bliss, aloof to the manifestation of the universe. Conceptualized as masculine, Shiva has all the power to be, but no power to manifest. The word *Shiva* in Sanskrit is a combined word: *Shava* means "dead" but the letter "i" makes it

Shiva. Without Shakti, Shiva is dead and cannot manifest anything. Neither Shiva nor Shakti can exist without the other. Although these two are inseparably united, in the manifested world there is an illusion of separation between pure consciousness and its manifestation. Shakti, the other part of the polarity, is the great mother of the universe because it is from her that all forms and names manifest. Shakti is a projection of consciousness that veils the pure consciousness from which she was projected. *Shakti* means "power or potential." However, only a small part of the energy of Shakti is involved in the manifestation of the world, while the greater part remains dormant.

The universal soul manifests with the help of the primal fire called kundalini shakti. Here, shakti is referred to as fire. This is not the fire that is used for digesting or cooking food, but the fire that is a direct power from the universal soul. The divine mother in you, who has given you all that you have, is direct shakti. This great fire manifests thousands of hot sparks that share its nature because they have all come out of the same cause, which in this instance is fire. There cannot be any cold sparks. Just as the sparks come out of the fire and again go back to it, the manifold world evolves from the indestructible and is again absorbed back into it. The sun without light is not the sun. Though the sun is different from its light, yet they are one and the same. The sun cannot exist without atma shakti. If there is no atma shakti, it is not atma.

THE POWER THAT MAKES A HUMAN BEING

All power comes from the center of consciousness. In the beginning in the vast ocean of bliss, there was silent movement *(satyam shivam sundaram)*, and from that silent movement the universe manifested. All of the five kingdoms—Monera, Protista, plants, fungi, animals—have evolved from the same source. From that first silent movement bubbles or sparks of Atman that would become individual souls emerged. The dynamic aspect of energy that provides the working force for the body and mind has evolved from Shakti and the primary most basic form of this energy within the human being is prana, which literally means the "first unit of life." PRANA IS THE SOURCE OF LIFE, the source of all manifestation. This sevenfold prana, this shakti, is capable of projecting the power of the individual soul. That is how it becomes individual. They are not individual as yet because they are still part of the ocean; they become individual only when *prana*, the life force, comes forward to create mind (unconscious and conscious), all the senses and the elements (space, air, fire, water and earth) that support the whole world, the two breaths and the body, which is made up of the five elements. To summarize, in the process of evolution, first the bubble comes, then the life energy and then the mind, breath and body. Prana is not the breath. When the seer of the Mundaka Upanishad described the sevenfold pranas, he was not talking about the breath. Prana rides the breath like a horse to reach the different parts of your system to energize them. Of course, THERE IS SOME FORCE THAT IS DIRECTING THE PRANA, otherwise it would just be dead air blowing from one part to another.

There is a difference between yogic and anatomical descriptions. Anatomy describes in minute detail all the parts that make up the physical body. Yoga science has thoroughly studied prana, the way it functions and the channels it uses. Yogic descriptions are used for the subtler energy levels and the prana that flows through the nadis or energy channels. Yoga science says there are thousands of vehicles that supply energy to various parts of your body.

According to the yoga manuals, there are 72,000 nadis. If one particular vehicle is not supplying energy properly, there will be pain, decay, abnormal growths such as malignant tumors, loss of function or deformity. As you have accidents in the external world, likewise when the nadis become congested, there are internal accidents that only a yogi can understand. Cancer is lack of control of yourself and your mind. This means a disease like cancer could be prevented if you learned how to use the energy vehicles and the mind.

Prana is not the kundalini. Prana is a different power that functions on multi levels called sheaths or *koshas.* The sheaths are: *annamaya kosha* (physical body or food sheath), *pranamaya* kosha (pranic sheath), *manomaya* kosha (mental sheath), *vijnanamaya* kosha (the buddhi or higher intellect) and *anandamaya* kosha (sheath of bliss). Physical energy is different, pranic energy is different, mental energy is different, and certainly, energy that is beyond mind, is different.

Prana makes up the PRANIC SHEATH that connects the body to the mind. Thus, the body mind relationship comes from prana, not from the kundalini. Likewise, the power to move does not come from the kundalini. Prana is described as flowing like a current through a series of subtle pathways (nadis) that connect the body and mind and help to coordinate body and mind functioning. On the more subtle third level of the sheaths prana is called mind, (MANAS). So the energy behind the thought process is also not due to the kundalini. Prana on the fourth level is the BUDDHI, or higher intellect as translated in English. There is, however, a difference between these two words. Buddhi is that faculty through which you gain internal and external knowledge; intellect is only related to knowing the facts with the help of the senses. The limitation of intellect is that intellect cannot go beyond the objective world. Neither supernatural experiences nor the experience of samadhi are within the realm of the intellect. Though there is something beyond intellect, intellect has its own power. When you lead your intellect with the help of facts, intellect decides, judges and discriminates. However, if you have not trained your intellect, then you cannot develop your awareness. On the fifth level prana is bliss (ANANDA).

If you really want to understand the sheaths properly, you have to understand their relationships and how they interact. Consciousness is often compared to a light, and the different sheaths are like lampshades that cover it. Due to the shades the light will appear to be very dim and the room will remain dark. These shades represent the limitations of the mind. You will have to remove the shades one by one until finally you will find the real light. These shades are made of different material, color and qualities. Each shade reflects light to a certain degree and modifies it according to its properties. The outermost shade is the densest one, so only a dim light can come through. As you remove each of them, the light becomes brighter. Because of the way these bodies conceal the light of consciousness, they are termed as sheaths or coverings. The moment you have destroyed all the superimpositions and have removed all the coverings of the lamp, the light will be there. Similarly, if you really want to know who you are, you have to remove all the masks, one after the other.

The sheaths do not function independently; they have a meaningful relationship because they are connected and coordinated. These connections are maintained by the seven main chakras. Without the kundalini shakti, it would not be possible for all the sheaths to remain connected.

As electrical energy is more subtle than mechanical energy, pranic energy is more subtle than electrical energy. You can continue to live even with very little prana. Even though you might appear to be physically and legally dead, you may still be alive.

Somehow two brothers in India learned this technique and started a business. One posed like a dead man, while the other told people his brother had died. The doctor came and confirmed he was dead. Then he would collect money because he would say he had no money to cremate his poor brother. The next day they would go to a different place. Once I was in the town where they were enacting their scheme. The people in the town told me that the doctor had pronounced this man dead. I asked them to bring a thermometer so I could insert it in the rectum. Immediately that "dead" brother came to life. They were using a simple technique of suspension of breath to fool everyone.

Prana, apana, vyana, udana and *samana* are the vehicles that prana uses. There are many vehicles and they do their work separately. For example, the sevenfold pranas that reside in the cave of the heart, provide the impetus for the growth of a human being. They are called sevenfold for the seven stages you pass through in your lifetime:

first, you are born; second, you become a child; third, you become an adult; fourth, you grow more to a stage of manhood or womanhood; fifth, you become a semi-old person; sixth, you become an old person and seventh, you go to death. Death is actually a part of growth. Have you seen a blue child? A blue child is one that has a hole in one of the chambers in the heart. As a result, arteries and veins communicate as one. This means the blood is not purified, so the growth of the child will be stunted. If you understand the channels of energy that reside in the cavity of the heart, then you will know those same channels exist in the universe, because the body is a miniature universe.

These sevenfold pranas are responsible to manifest themselves in multitudinous ways. That's why there are mountains, rivers, forests and everything else in the universe. Innumerable illusory manifestations, *(maya),* bring forth the universe. After eons of time when the universe will be dissolved, it will be drawn back into Shakti, the same source that is the basis of its manifestation. There is actually no difference between the universe of forms and names and the universe without forms and names. The manifested one and the unmanifested are one reality.

THREE SELVES

Actually, you are three selves: mortal, semi-immortal and immortal. The body, the breath and the conscious mind make up the mortal self or the small self. The semi-immortal part is the unconscious mind where you store all the samskaras or impressions of all your life experiences. It is the bed of memory or storehouse of merits and demerits. You have desires to fulfill and it is those desires that have motivated you to project forward.

In this way the unconscious has a vehicle and a force. That's how it has become individual. It becomes perfectly immortal when it drops these superimpositions. For example, *I have a body* is an imposition. When you talk of the immortal Self, you are talking of the real Self.

THE EVOLUTION OF SPIRITUALITY

Now, from the absolute One also came forward the mantras of the *Rigveda, Samaveda, Atharvaveda* and *Yajurveda.* The Vedas are said to be ancient scriptures. Westerners are confused because the same Vyasa that compiled the Vedas was also the author of the Mahabharata. They wonder how one man could have lived for so many generations. The answer is Vyasa was not a person. Just as the Himalayan Institute is an institute and not a person, in the same manner, Vyasa is like the name of an institute. One after another there was a lineage where scholars did the same work under the name of Vyasa. If Swami Rama goes away, another swami will teach you the same things. Therefore, the date cannot be set when the Vedas first came into existence. Knowledge is knowledge; nobody has created it. It is eternal, whether it has come from the Christian Bible or the Vedas or any other source. KNOWLEDGE IS ALWAYS ETERNAL BECAUSE ULTIMATELY IT HAS COME FROM THE ABSOLUTE ONE.

VEDAS

According to Vedic science, there are four ages on earth: *Satya Yug, Treta Yug, Dwapara Yug* and the present *Kali Yug.* During Satya Yug, no one spoke lies because no one knew anything but truth, and everyone was in bliss. The ancient seers of the Vedic Age, Satya Yug, were far superior to the *avatars* (incarnate divine teachers).

Any knowledge that came from the avatars was indirect knowledge *(smriti)*. On the other hand, the seers received direct knowledge *(shruti)*. The great sages and the great prophets all received that wisdom from within, from the center of consciousness from where consciousness is flowing on various degrees and grades. *Revelation* is "knowledge that flows from the library of the eternal." The knowledge of the seers has not come through the senses or the mind, but rather it has come through visions. Those visions were based on self-evident knowledge that does not need support or any evidence. When you receive a vision you see things as they are, not as you want them to be. In order to see things as they are, you will have to reach the top of the mountain from where you can see the valley, what is to the right and the left of the valley and what is beyond. The sages discovered several methods to accomplish this.

Later, Indian communities started to worship avatars such as Rama and Krishna because they did not know how to study or practise the ancient wisdom of the Vedas. No doubt Rama and Krishna were great men, but they could not compare with the seers. Since they could not give anything new to the world, they modified the philosophy of the ancient seers. The knowledge I am presenting to you has not come through my mind. A bit of it is has come through visions and the rest from the teachings of the great ones whom I had the privilege of living with and enjoying their love and blessings.

In Treta Yug, the next cycle, people started to perform *yagyas* (in Hinduism, a ritual with fire) and degeneration came. In Treta Yug they only did chanting, but in Dwapara Yug they included many other practices. In both Treta and Dwapara they performed *agni yagyas* to kill the animal in human beings so they could realize they were spiritual beings. You are a compound of three: animal, human, and divine. The animal in the human being does not want to be disciplined. The more the animal nature is active in your life, the more difficult it is to be disciplined. The human in the human being wants to be disciplined when they have had a glimpse of knowledge of the absolute. Although a fortunate few were wise and became realized, most of them could not attain the absolute reality. And so, spirituality, instead of going through a final filtration, slowly went to the gutters and there was overall degeneration of humanity. It is up to you to seek the prestige and dignity of your true Self, so that even now in Kali Yug where the mind of human beings is dissipated and scattered, you can realize.

PATANJALI'S YOGA SUTRAS

A few centuries before Christ, the great sage Patanjali systematized and organized the study of the internal states of mind and consciousness in a series of aphorisms called the Yoga Sutras. *Sutra* means "string." An *aphorism* is a concise statement of a general principle or truth. Because they are so concise, they must be expanded in order to be understood. If you read the Yoga Sutras without guidance, you will become more confused. This means the sutras are not meant for a confused person because they can create more confusion.

It is very interesting how one aphorism is related to another. In those aphorisms you will find not only science, yoga techniques and philosophy but also psychology. I studied the Yoga Sutras many times in my childhood, yet I still did not know much about them. There are 196 aphorisms in the Yoga Sutras, which have been divided into four sections or *padas:* In the first pada, *Samadhi Pada,* Patanjali has explained that mind and its modifications have to be under your control. In *Sadhana Pada,* the second pada, Patanjali has given the practical aspects of the Yoga Sutras as the first five steps of Ashtanga Yoga. In *Vibhuti Pada,* the third pada, Patanjali describes *samyama,* the process of inner transformation that leads to enlightenment, the highest state of wisdom and bliss, which in turn leads to the acquisition of special spiritual powers *(siddhis).* Patanjali describes how siddhis can be attained and how to perform miracles. These simply involve higher techniques that you do not know, so you call them miracles. Christ knew the techniques, but his guru John the Baptist, did not know. You can know something that your guru does not know. Christ came in touch with those powers because he knew more about mind and its potentials. That's why he was able to change water into wine. Miracles are miracles as long as you do not understand them. The moment you understand them, they are no longer miracles. The fourth pada is *Kaivalya,* the final stage or liberation.

YOGA SCIENCE AND YOGA PSYCHOLOGY

The word *psychology* means "the science of mental life." But modern psychology has not yet developed to the extent where it can claim it knows how to study all aspects of mental life. Modern or Western psychology did not come about by studying the thinking process or because of the prime necessity of realization, but rather it came about by studying behavior, and is therefore based on behaviorism. However, very little of the mind is expressed through behavior, so you cannot study the totality of mind simply by studying behavior.

How to apply yoga science to know your Self is called yoga psychology, which is the very foundation of Eastern or ancient psychology. Although yoga psychology is very deep, it can be understood only by practising it, not by memorizing the aphorisms of the Yoga Sutras. Patanjali says first you have to go to the deeper levels of your being and understand your internal states. Through the Yoga Sutras he leads you on an inward journey by first making you aware of all the functions and various faculties of the mind. Those faculties of mind are creating obstacles for you because you are trying to search for enlightenment in the external world. That is not the way.

SCIENCE OF SELF-DEVELOPMENT

Life is divided into two aspects: life within and life without. Meditation helps you to understand both aspects and provides a bridge to the other shore, the unknown part of your life. You are on a journey that goes from gross to subtle, to the subtler and then the most subtle aspect of your life. You can be lost in the external world because there are many distractions. On the contrary, it's very easy to find within because there are less disturbances from the external world. You don't lose anything in meditation and you never become insane when you practise meditation. You are comfortable with the known but you fear the unknown. Sooner or later you will have to become familiar with your thinking process and samskaras, so don't be afraid of that. In meditation you come in touch with a part of yourself you have not known before. Naturally, it will give you some jolts. When you understand your relationship with the external world and learn to deal with it, the waking reality and its distractions will no longer create new grooves in your mind and heart. Then, the path of the Self becomes simple and your desires will start to flow inward instead of to the external world. This is your birth right. However, you cannot live within only. You have to create a bridge between within and without. The outside world gives you the means to satisfy and help that part of life that needs comfort.

It is unfortunate that there is no definite training program that would facilitate knowledge of the internal states. Without knowing one's inner dimensions, one remains a stranger to oneself. Education encourages the examination and verification only of external objects, but human potential cannot be explored by exploring the external world. This is why it is important to impart the knowledge of understanding oneself in childhood, so that every child understands themself as a nucleus and the world around them as its expansion. The seeds that are sown in childhood have a deep impact and impression on the mind and the emotional nature. Unfortunately, from your childhood onward you have been taught to see and examine things in the external world and to be very active and efficient in your work, but no one has taught you to be still, to search within and verify within. This very essential part of life has been totally ignored by the educational system. It is essential to provide to your children an education that is holistically complete and helps them to know their inner life as well. A definite method should become a part of the educational curriculum so that from the beginning every child understands their potential and develops sensitivity for others. When children realize everyone breathes one and the same breath no matter from which country or cultural background they come, then there will be peace, understanding and equilibrium in the world. Peace is a relative term. A gap between two wars is called peace in the world. But that is not what you want. You want peace that lasts as long as you live.

The one-sided education that is imparted in the colleges and universities is imperfect and incomplete and helps one only to earn a livelihood rather than to develop awareness of the Self within. This is why violence, conflicts and chaos are rampant in modern society. Conflict within and without is the arch enemy that separates one human being from other human beings. These conflicts arise from the ego and selfishness because human beings are not taught to be genuine, loving, sharing and caring in their childhood. All conflicts in society, in the family and within your own self, exist because you do not know yourself on all levels. Today, you may think you have known something after attending a seminar, after talking to a teacher or after reading a book. But there is no end as far as knowledge is concerned. You have made many efforts to be successful in the world, but you haven't made any effort to know yourself. If you really want to know yourself you should first examine the situation in which you live. In the world you may have a good home and family, good relationships, enough to spend and prestige. You have many means, all that you need in your daily life, yet you are not happy. You need to apply all that you have for something higher. You should try to study your internal states for a few minutes every day. I am not going to accept the excuse that you don't have time. You have time to eat, drink and enjoy, so why can't you have time to study your internal states? All your actions in the external world are controlled and commanded from within. Then why are you not trying to understand that there is something within you that is responsible for all your activities and that should also be understood? Meditation is not a religion or a game, but something very helpful and useful in daily life. It is not only the mere study of your internal states but something that makes your mind tranquil, relaxes your body and nervous system and helps you to know more about yourself. The more you know yourself, the more you can know others. This is very helpful in family life, in married life, in friendship and also in daily actions and duties.

In modern society the idea of developing human potential is a frequent topic of discussion and study, yet very little is known about the extent of that potential. This is because nowhere in society is it possible to comprehensively study the true nature of human potential and the methods by which that potential can unfold. Similarly, even the sciences of self-development suggest an equally clouded perspective when it comes to understanding the possibility of fuller mental potential. In fact, abstract intellectual knowledge is emphasized at the expense of more meaningful and more powerful ways of knowing. Current circumstances reveal untrained minds that are subject to the influence of indiscriminate foods and other substances that dull consciousness and make the mind operate sluggishly and without clarity. On the other hand, minds that remain distracted and agitated from overstimulation are scattered and chaotic. Further, there is very little understanding of the personality and the emotional level of human experience or of the extent of human beings' ability to develop their fullest potential.

Human beings are still in the process of evolution. Despite the work of Jung, Maslow and others who have tried to explore what lies beyond the most primitive levels of the human personality, we often cannot even agree on what the most evolved characteristics of human personality are. What would a human being be like who was not depressed, anxious or angry, who was not troubled by insecurity, loneliness or conflicts? How would such a person behave in relation to both themself and others? Would such persons be satisfied with the quest for mundane wealth, fame and pleasure that occupies most of our waking attention, or are there other more powerful forces that would motivate them? Here, too, our experience may have led us to become imbalanced because so often we have found that those who claim to have developed more fully or to be more actualized are in fact struggling with the same insecurities and selfishness from which most human beings suffer. As a result, many people may decide simply to give up the whole question of how to develop their personality or unfold their highest potential. Without a map of the direction of development or how to achieve it, there is no real hope that such a transformation is even possible. Most therapies and therapists do not themselves understand the full potential of human beings. Instead, they focus on a sense of negativity and inadequacy, and have few tools to help students and patients move beyond their limited potential to an experience of greater health, peace and joy.

Recently, however, in new areas of research, medicine and therapy, there has been an interest in more fully understanding human potential. For example, some human beings have the ability to heal apparent diseases in themselves or to express potentials that others find difficult even to imagine. These subtle and inspiring abilities have long been understood and acknowledged within meditative traditions. While many sceptics and those who are afraid may scoff, there are numerous examples of individuals whose powers of understanding and control of the body have led them to amazing feats that are not the result of mere deception or trickery, but represent instead a genuine understanding of the human vehicle on much deeper levels than that exhibited by most human beings.

How to cultivate or consciously develop the potentials of mind is generally not known. Mind has vast potentials that can be utilized, such as creativity, intuition and insight that are far beyond the normal levels of functioning. These levels usually remain blocked because human beings primarily devote their energy and time to pursuing their own shallow individual desires, thus preventing them from unfolding their personality and expanding their consciousness. But when a human being begins to open up to life in a different way, expanding their ability to love and accept others, then these higher aspects of mind and personality become available. In short, it is the selfishness and self-centeredness of human beings that is the main barrier to the expression and experience of these innate, higher potentials.

In contrast to this state of affairs, the ancient sciences of human consciousness and development have explored and described in great detail the possibilities of human potential. In fact, they offer a comprehensive and systematic program based on the primary assumption that the unfolding of this potential is the central goal and responsibility of every human being, and that all have the possibility of realizing their essential nature. Meditation and the development of the personality lead to such a state that allows for the experience of this potential. The system of meditation considers these higher potentials to be only the beginning of the process. The final goal is the experience of the highest state of human potential, a state in which the human being recognizes the transcendence and perfection in all things to experience truth, unity and the highest joy within, and the recognition of this essence in others. This is the ultimate potential of human beings and it lies within. It is the birth right and essential nature of all human beings. The reality is a vast part of your life but unfortunately it remains unknown. You have hidden the finest part of yourself because you don't know anything about it. If you want to know the unknown just be calm and allow the unknown to come forward. Don't create obstacles for yourself. You should enjoy every second of life by understanding the real goal of life. All of the things of the world are your means; you should apply those means to attain that goal.

CONSCIOUSNESS and HUMAN POTENTIAL

CONSCIOUSNESS
STATES of CONSCIOUSNESS
GOD
PURPOSE of LIFE
SADHANA

CONSCIOUSNESS

If you carefully examine the human being in its totality you will find that individual existence is more than matter, energy and mind. According to the ancient spiritual traditions, the basic principle of the Self or pure consciousness underlies all of these and is the ultimate experience of human potential. Consciousness is described as ever pure, ever wise and ever free. Consciousness is always with you no matter where you move, though you are not aware of it because of mind's limitations. When you go to the center of consciousness, you will not find mind there. Ordinarily, you have no awareness of the Self and instead define yourself in ways that emphasize your limitations and imperfections. Thus, because you do not know the highest Self, you feel insecure and become depressed with your apparent limitations in body, mind and personality. So far, there have been many experiments on the body, on energy and on some aspects of mind, but human potential actually resides in the center of consciousness. Though there is only one consciousness flowing, it flows through many avenues. Similarly, there are various levels of enlightenment and also various levels of ignorance. For example, I see you so I am conscious that you exist. But this does not enlighten me or you. Then, another level of consciousness comes in which you recognize that other human beings are just like you, so you should not hurt anyone. Still there is another level in which you realize you have no right to hurt anyone because you actually would be hurting yourself. As you progress, you become more aware of the reality until gradually you get freedom from the bondages you have been creating because of ignorance. IGNORANCE IS THE MOTHER OF ALL PROBLEMS.

Consciousness, the center of the life force within you, is not in the body, because the body changes, grows and finally goes to death, decay and destruction. Likewise, it is not in the breath, the senses or the thinking process. Even when the body falls apart, the loss of body consciousness does not affect you. You can voluntarily withdraw your mind from body consciousness and divert it to the center of consciousness within. Everyone does not have access to the center of consciousness because of lack of preparation and awareness. If you can you attain that state where you don't have body, breath, senses and mind consciousness, you will be there.

Consciousness is not in the external world or in the dreaming world. It is beyond all that. CONSCIOUSNESS IS WITHIN YOU. Therefore, learn to go to the deeper aspects of your being, the source of life and light, pure consciousness. You have that power. When one seeks self-transformation and undertakes the process of perfecting the personality and moving away from depression, selfishness and anger, then one begins a process by which consciousness begins to unfold and express itself on all degrees and levels. These deeper, subtle potentials and powers of the human being are nothing like the sensational and egotistical demonstrations of human beings who seek attention, fame and material gain by using particular abilities to entertain and impress others.

STATES OF CONSCIOUSNESS

A sadhaka who is aware of the many levels of consciousness starts to question life and to examine all the levels of life, including the different states of consciousness. STATES OF CONSCIOUSNESS ARE ENTIRELY DIFFERENT FROM STATES OF MIND. States of mind are related only to the thinking process and the emotions. For example, feeling pain and pleasure are states of mind. On the other hand, states of consciousness are fields of the activities of the external world: THE WAKING STATE, THE DREAMING STATE, THE SLEEPING STATE AND TURIYA. They are not states of mind, creations of the mind or projections of the mind.

Whatsoever is seen here, there and everywhere is Brahman. There is no place where there is not Brahman or the ultimate reality. Atman verily is Brahman and has four aspects. The first aspect is the waking state or *vaishwanara*. When consciousness is turned to the external world, this is the waking state. The conscious mind is used only during the waking state. The moment you wake up in the morning, your conscious mind immediately starts to use the senses. Actually, the conscious mind is always controlled by the greater part of mind. Human beings have not yet understood the right utilization of the waking state, and there is no university that teaches you how to dream. As a result, when you are in the sleeping state or dreaming state, a vast part of the mind remains unknown to you. Therefore, you cannot cultivate the dreaming and sleeping states as long as they remain unknown to you. Since you do not know much about the different states of consciousness, this means you know very little about yourself. As a result, your intelligence is limited to only one aspect of the totality of the learning process. During the waking and dreaming states, your mind and senses are not under your control, but you can learn how to have control over them. There are techniques that can help you to know the condition of your mind in all three states. This will lead to the next state, the fourth state of turiya.

To begin, who experiences these states? You say: *I* experienced the waking state, *I* dreamt, *I* slept. Who is that *I* who remains fully awake while you were in deep sleep, when you were dreaming or when you were fully awake? It means there is someone beyond all these three states that remains fully awake. Actually, consciousness, the Atman or THE INDIVIDUAL SOUL IS THE ONE THAT EXPERIENCES THE THREE STATES, because mind does not have the capacity to do that. When the individual soul experiences vaishwanara (waking state), it experiences the gross world and the external objects of the world. The one that experiences the waking state is the same that experiences *tejasa* (dreaming state), *pragya* (sleeping state) and whose permanent abode is turiya. Consciousness experiences the different states of waking, dreaming, and sleeping; ETERNITY REMAINS EVER AWAKE. What is the difference between the dreaming and the waking state? As you say, this all appears to be true, and the dreaming state is also true as long as it lasts. When you are in deep sleep, nothing is true. But if you go to turiya, you will find that TURIYA ALONE IS TRUTH.

Then the question comes, where do you exist? As a human being, your consciousness, your individual soul exists in the waking, dreaming or sleeping states, but you actually dwell in the fourth state, turiya. Your duty is to establish the supreme *I* in place of the little *I* (ego), because ego has separated you from the whole. The method of meditation will help you, but you will have to include *vichara* (contemplation) and you will also have to learn to have an inner dialogue (discussed in section on Mind and Meditation). Inner dialogue is like a form of self-psychiatry.

Dreams are very good for your mental health because they provide an emotional outlet. But if you know the method of allowing your mind to go through a process faster than dream, you can dream two years' dream in one day. You can even dream your whole life's dream in one day. It is even possible to give a dream to a friend while they are sleeping, no matter where they are, but this cannot happen with a stranger. And it will only work when they are fast asleep and the conscious mind has calmed down. During that time you can send your thought forms, and it will be very easy for them to receive them. You should sit down at two o'clock in the morning while your friend is sleeping and mentally send your thought forms. Their sleep will be disturbed, and if you do it over and over, they will have a dream. I have examined this many times. If you know the method of how to allow the entire unconscious mind to come forward to the conscious level, you can dream everything, because this is all just a dream. The great sages understood that the world is not the truth. TRUTH IS BEYOND THIS DREAM.

GOD

In the West and in Christian religions, the absolute reality (Brahman) or pure consciousness is referred to as *God*. They are one and the same. Just like Brahman, God is omnipresent, omniscient and omnipotent. Since God is everywhere, there is no space for God to move, so there cannot be two gods. If you ask a Western child where is God, the child will point to the sky, but an Eastern child will point to the heart. Both are right. God doesn't just exist beyond the clouds; God is there and here both because GOD IS EVERYWHERE. God does not exist only in a statue, on a rock or on the mountains but is especially present in everyone's spiritual heart, the center of the life force within you. It is beyond body, breath, senses and mind. If God is omnipresent, you should not say He is only up there. He is everywhere, or He is not God. If you think

God is a little bit there, a little bit here and a little bit in me, then you are talking about something else, but not God. You cannot cut God into pieces and say a little bit of God is in Swami Rama, and a big part of God is in the universe. It is very easy to think God exists somewhere far away, and you are small and good for nothing. If you are not aware of the reality within you, you will remain ignorant and you will lose self-confidence. When you believe God is far away from you, you don't feel safe and you don't have self-confidence. Those who are not conscious of the eternal stream of life remain under the fear of death and do not enjoy life. All your worries exist because you don't have faith that the Lord is in you. Because God is omnipresent, omniscient and omnipotent, God is in everyone. It is not possible that anyone could be excluded.

Even though you feel inspired when you remember that Christ could see God, still you have the desire to see God with your two eyes without having any concept or understanding of what God is. What do you mean when you say you want to see God? The language you are using is not accurate. You say the sun rises in the East and sets in the West, even though you understand the sun never actually rises or sets. The sun is always there; it is the earth that is moving. You think for something to exist you have to be able to see it with your eyes. If somebody is blind, does it mean that person will never see God? If God exists everywhere, you want to see and touch God. You chant the name of God, you study books about God and you say you want to see God but you have not decided what you expect from God. If you do not know God is within and you are still searching for God outside, there is something wrong. If you cannot find God within how do you expect to find God outside? You have to get rid of that confusion and be at peace so you can realize the great glory that is hidden deep in your heart. There was a time when I also used to think that I should see God during meditation and I used to cry and weep about it. When my master asked me what I expected from God, I finally realized I shouldn't expect anything from God but instead I should expect something from myself. I came to understand I had to explore and understand the various dimensions of my life. So, before you try to understand what God is, you should understand yourself.

All the things in the world have some name and form. There is no form that does not go to change, death and decay. Name and form are only temporary aspects of something that goes on changing. When you identify yourself with the external world that is constantly changing, you become sad. You condemn yourself because you identify with the body that is perishable. You are attached to the perishable because you have forgotten your true nature. You are committing a serious mistake, whether you are meditating or not, by being so attached to your body that you think your body is your greatest friend. But the body is very weak. Sometimes it functions well and sometimes it doesn't. To rely on a friend that is very weak and not always a fit instrument is not good. You should observe and understand your relationship with the body. You are not the body; the body is different from you. In this lifetime, you should attain that state of freedom where you can voluntarily dissociate yourself from body consciousness. Many meditators knowingly and consciously can free themselves from body consciousness and can see themselves outside their body. It is better to rely upon and identify with the source within that gives strength to the body. You cannot know that source through the mind, because it is beyond mind. It would be better to surrender yourself to the source within. When you start to do meditation, you will find that your greatest friend is within.

Whomever you call God or absolute truth is not far away from you, so there is no need to try to see God. When your whole being becomes an eye you will see God. You should have confidence that the Lord of life is within you. God, Atman, is within you and you are that Atman. THOU ART THAT. If He is in you, He is in you with all His majesty. Knowing this will give you great confidence and you will be fearless. Confidence comes when you go to the source that is the immortal part of your being. When you understand that God is within, you will always be with God and you will feel safe. The more you become aware of the reality within you, the more confident you will become. There is no point in having confidence in the body, senses or mind because they are subject to change, death and decay. That which does not have its own existence cannot give you confidence. You should have confidence in Atman, the cosmic soul. When you say you are different from God you are insulting the Lord who exists everywhere. There is no need to wait for God to come down to you or to wait for your next life to know God. God is not something external to you. The best part of you is God, the reality that is truth and is not subject to change, death or decay. Such a great friend you have, that is very strong, everlasting and full of peace and bliss. And you are ignoring it and instead giving the most importance to the body, which is only weak flesh that will decay and decompose. You have to remember you are not limited to body or mind alone. You are very great, but you know only a small part of yourself. THE GREATEST AND BEST PART OF YOU IS GOD; the lowest part is the body. You know only your body so you think you are the body, but the day that you understand that God, the power of powers, is within you, you will be free from limitations.

Some of you say you don't believe in God. God has never asked you to believe in Him. If you don't believe in the sun, even then the sun will still shine for you; if you don't believe in the breeze, still you will get air. However, if you believe in God, you will have to accept that God is within. You should learn to pray to and be in communion with the One who is directly within you and who is the very essence of life. When you come to know that God dwells in you, then your life and concept of life will totally change and you will be transformed. You will no longer feel your individual existence. If God is in you, it means you are a living shrine of God. You should look after this shrine knowing it is the Lord's shrine. The greatest of all wonders in the world is that this finite vessel that ultimately will go to change, death and decay carries something infinite. God walks with you, witnesses all your actions and purifies your soul, which is part of the ultimate truth. I rarely speak in temples because according to my philosophy, every human being is a temple. If I do not see God in you and then go to the temple and search for God there, I am not being faithful to my Lord. There is no temple that is higher than you. Deep within you is the fountain of life and light. When you come in touch with that part of your life, you will be free. You are not as small as you think you are. Human potentials are immense. You are great because God, the highest of all truths, dwells within you. YOU ARE IN GOD, GOD IS IN YOU. Your whole being exists because of God who is giving you the power to speak, to hear and to think. If you really believe in God and you are in search of God, you will have to become aware of this reality. But for lack of Self-realization, you suffer. You have to realize yourself before you meet the Self of all. You do not need to retire from the world or go to a Himalayan retreat to realize the Self. The greatest miracle is that infinity dwells in you, a finite vessel. Knowing that, you should feel great joy and have great confidence. Instead, you are carrying the infinite within and moaning around because your mind has created a barrier between you and the infinite. You need to work with your mind and your samskaras from the unconscious so you can become bold and courageous. Every individual should try to know themself on all levels and have the determination to be enlightened here and now.

From morning until evening, where is the place for God in your daily life and what is the purpose of God in your daily life? There are things you have been repeating without understanding why you are doing them. This sort of faith is better than not being conscious and not having faith, but it doesn't help much. If God is everywhere, God is in you. You have simply to go deep inside to where that center of silence resides with all its glory. SEE GOD WITHIN. You can converse directly with God. God is talking through you, seeing through you and listening through you. God exists everywhere so He exists outside too. But here, you are trying to meditate, which is an inward method. In that method your very desire is to meet God who is within you. You sit down and you say, *I will see God as I see things outside; I will even see God clearly in me. But my eyes are closed, so I cannot see with my eyes. I will have to open the eye of my mind and make my whole being an eye so I can truly see.* What I see through my mind when I am in meditation is much clearer than what I can see through my eyes.

No matter how much you sharpen your conscious mind or how many books you study you are training only a small part of mind. Human potentials and resources are immense, but you do not know how to use them. You have to go to the infinite library within and bring forth that knowledge to be creative in the external world. Nothing is impossible. You can do anything if you really know the source that is within you. You have all the powers within you, but you have no faith in yourself. If you do not have faith in yourself, how can you have faith in God? To develop faith in God first you have to have faith in yourself and your own existence. Then you will have to understand the existence of the universe. For that you have to learn how to be still and go within yourself.

Self-confidence is very essential, but it is also essential to take help from the transpersonal mind rather than always from the small personal mind. The transpersonal field is not the field of ordinary knowledge. You have to know the method of how to access transpersonal knowledge. It is dangerous to rely on the intellect all the time or to be swayed by the emotions. You will have to work with these two. Emotions can drive you crazy. As long as you are using your intellect you are not tapping the source of inner knowledge. The intellect can make you very egotistical and you will never learn because ego creates a barrier between you and transpersonal knowledge. Ego makes you believe you already know everything, so there is no need to know anything else. You often pray to God to help you remove all obstacles. If you think you can go on creating misery for yourself because God will remove it, that is never going to happen. You all have God's grace but you are miserable because you don't have your own grace! Fifty per cent of grace is dependent on your actions, and fifty per cent is already there. You are not aware of two powers. One power is the ascending force that depends on human effort. When you have made human effort, then you receive a blessing that is called the descending force. Human effort is the greatest of all virtues. You don't get anything without doing an action. Therefore, don't think that without human effort you will ever attain peace, happiness and wisdom. Human misery comes first from conflict within and without; second, from lack of contentedness regarding one's self; and third, from fear of the unknown. The finest philosophy is one that helps you to realize that God is in every human being and that human beings are the most evolved beings in the world and the finest of all species on earth. If you learn to explore all the different levels of consciousness, you can finally go to the highest center of awareness.

PURPOSE OF LIFE

There are three categories of people. TIME-ORIENTED people are those who are concerned about tomorrow and what is going to happen in the next moment. They say they want to live *now*, even though they don't understand what *now* means. Another category is GOAL-ORIENTED people who have material goals in life and are considered to be successful in the world. They are educated and have status, enough means and all the necessary amenities of life. And the final category is PURPOSE-ORIENTED people whose predominant concern is to attain the purpose of life. All human beings have the right to attain the final goal of life and to understand the mystery of life and the purpose of life, but it is not easy. The first thing you need to remember is that you are here for a brief period of time and eventually you will have to leave. Many of you think you have come to this world to remain forever, and so you have become irresponsible and have forgotten the purpose of life. That is why it is important to make the best use of this opportunity, no matter from which culture, religion or philosophical background you have come. Whatever you do, wherever you go, you should always remember the goal of life. Many people say the goal of life is to know God, but they cannot explain what it means to know God. Nothing happens if you don't know God. Even if one tiny little bit of you remembers God, nothing will happen to God, nor will you become the jewel in God's crown. If you are aware of the reality all the time, then all your activities will be motivated toward truth. Once you understand that life is not merely relating to people and accumulating many things you will come to realize that life has a deeper purpose.

It is not possible to make the physical body immortal, although it is possible to expand your lifespan and live for 100 or even 150 years. But I have not met anyone anywhere in the world who could keep the body forever. In this lifetime, you should learn the technique of using this instrument called body as much as you can for the purpose of life. And then, when this body falls apart, you should learn to withdraw your mind so that body consciousness does not affect you.

What is important is that you continue to work with yourself, no matter who you are. The thought, *I am going to enlighten myself,* should not make you egotistical and you should not isolate yourself. This thought should make you more creative, because to withdraw yourself from the world is not life's purpose. Your life's purpose is to live in the world and yet remain above it.

THE PURPOSE OF HUMAN LIFE IS TO ATTAIN A STATE OF PEACE, HAPPINESS AND WISDOM. When mind is in equilibrium, is not dissipated or agitated and there is no conflict, that orderly state is called PEACE. It means there is perfect coordination between the modifications of mind in your thinking, decisions and actions. This helps your mind to attain a state of equilibrium and tranquillity. Searching for peace and joy outside is like chewing a weed that has very little water content so it can never quench your thirst. YOU HAVE TO SEARCH FOR PEACE WITHIN YOURSELF. And once you have gained this inner peace, no outside circumstances can ever disturb you, even when you are fully engaged in action in the most difficult and complex situations.

Once, a horseman who was riding through a forest decided to stop at a nearby well because he was feeling tired and thirsty and he felt his horse must also be thirsty. Unfortunately, the mechanism that helps to draw water from the well was making a lot of noise, and that noise was very annoying. So, when the horseman tried to take his horse there, the horse naturally tried to run away. The horseman asked the man who was attending the well to stop the sound from coming, because it was scaring his horse.

The man replied, "If the sound stops, the water will also stop."

"What to do?" the horseman asked.

The other man replied, "Create a condition for your horse so that the horse will drink water in this situation."

Through sincere effort, you have to create such a condition in this world so you can live happily. Otherwise, the water will stop. You all want to stop the noise and the pollution, yet if you go to the forest where there is nothing, you will be disturbed by the rush and roar of the winds and the breeze. YOU CANNOT FIND PEACE ANYWHERE IF THERE IS NO PEACE WITHIN. Peace does not mean there should be no noise. The noise will continue, but still you should have peace within. In all situations, you should be peaceful, no matter what happens.

HAPPINESS is a state free from all pain and misery. It is not something you have to gain; happiness is your true nature. Though you are running around, making effort and working hard, you may also lie, cheat and do many things to enter into the competition that modern society has created to attain so-called happiness. And still you are not happy. This means you are not properly applying your means toward your goal. Mind has the habit to run here and there, so it is difficult to understand, think or perceive anything accurately. You become lost in the world and forget your aim in life. Any action you are performing should be to have happiness and to know the ultimate truth and the purpose of life. You all are searching for that, some consciously and others not so consciously. This is difficult for you because the charms and temptations of the world are very powerful and they lead all of your attention to the external world and dissipate your energy. As you are searching, working and making effort for material goals, never forget that the center of happiness lies within you, not in the external world. THE OUTSIDE WORLD CANNOT BE AVOIDED, BUT IT HAS NEVER GIVEN TRUE HAPPINESS TO ANYBODY.

You are a citizen of two worlds, the world within and the world outside. Wise is the person who establishes a healthy link between these two worlds. You can run away from the world to escape or you can remain in the world with the fear you might lose what you have or you might not gain what you want. Life under these pressures becomes miserable. As long as the lake of the mind remains disturbed, there can be no happiness. When you are able to still the waves of the lake of the mind, you will find happiness within. If you live with light all the time, you will never be in the dark. Your true nature is happiness, but you create unhappiness for yourself. If you remain aware of the reality all the time, there can be no place for unhappiness in life. Never postpone happiness for tomorrow but just be happy all the time. Happiness means adjustment, which brings contentment. If you are able to adjust with all your relationships you will feel happy. If you do not have conflicts within you will not have conflicts outside. If you are free from conflicts within and without and free from misery and pain, you will be in a state of happiness. HAPPINESS IS A HIGHER LEVEL OF CONSCIOUSNESS THAT IS BEYOND PAIN AND PLEASURE.

As a human being you are fully equipped with the power and potential to remove all of the misery in your life, provided you know the methods of how to do so and you make sincere human effort. Even though you may be making efforts to attain a state of everlasting happiness, your desire is frequently intercepted by pain, misery and worry that come to you through bad food, wrong lifestyle or through not understanding the right course and conduct of life. You eat, drink and enjoy the things of the world without understanding why you are doing this. All human begins have the same rights to have enough to eat and live comfortably, but if you do not understand the purpose of life you will never be happy. You are all living, and want to live for a hundred years. Do you want to live for a hundred years just to enjoy the things of the world? You do not believe you are going to die. You see other people dying, but you don't see yourself dying. Death is terrifying to you, but do you feel that in your daily lives? You see that people die every day, but a part of you never dies, and you also feel that every day. If you go around thinking, *I will die just as my neighbor died!* then you will not be able to do anything in life. But if you understand the immortality within, then you will be very happy and there will be no fear.

You have known the quality and nature of the things that you have been enjoying and you think you cannot live without them. But you should be aware of their transitory nature. The senses come in touch with the external world with the help of mind and the energy that flows from the center of consciousness. This is not under your control. You are constantly contacting the objects of the world with the help of your senses. And when your senses contact matter, you receive one of two sensations — pain or pleasure. Being afraid of pain magnifies the pain. Mind should be kept pleasantly busy so that the feeling of pain could be lessened. You have to know how to consciously withdraw your senses. That is why in Ashtanga Yoga pratyahara is very important. There are books on concentration, meditation and samadhi, but there are no books on pratyahara because it's a practical technique. You have to learn to turn inward and withdraw your senses, because the senses are dragging you to the external world. That is why you feel pain and pleasure.

In *Mundaka Upanishad* there is a story of two birds in the tree of life, which has its roots above and branches going downward. One is constantly eating the fruits of this tree of life that are pleasant or unpleasant, that are fearful or full of sorrow, while the other is only witnessing. Pain and pleasure, two opposites, live together. One suffers, one enjoys. If you want to enjoy be prepared for suffering too, because the source of pleasure and pain is one and the same. They are identical companions, living on the same tree, very close to each other. One is called Brahman and the other is called jivatma. One is immortal and the other is also, but because of its superimpositions, and because of ignorance, it suffers. She suffers because she identifies with and has become entangled with external objects. Nobody has created any problems for the bird that is suffering; she has created her problems for herself. She simply has to change her attitude. The moment she recognizes the glory and greatness of the bird that is witnessing, she will attain freedom from all pain and misery.

You make effort to achieve things in the external world for happiness, but they only serve the purpose of giving you the means. The world can furnish all the means, but it cannot lead you to the goal of peace, happiness and wisdom. Even having the best means and all the pleasures of the world will not make you happy, because in addition you have to have the right attitude toward life. The right attitude is your mental outlook after having understood life and its purpose. You will have to learn to apply the means to attain everlasting happiness.

When you forget your aim and you do not know how to apply those means to attain happiness, those means will create obstacles for you. This is how that which gives you joy, which is a necessity and means for you, becomes an obstacle to happiness. In the comfortable life that you lead in the external world, those comforts have made you a slave because you have forgotten your real aim. No matter how much you search, there is nothing to grasp that can be called happiness. HAPPINESS IS A STATE THAT IS FREE FROM PAIN AND MISERY. You have created pain because of your ignorance, and because you do not study your own life process. If you talk to yourself in a balanced manner, that dialogue with the self will bring forward all your hidden frustrations and desires. If you are afraid to encounter your life, your thinking process, emotions and feelings will become stronger and will create many diseases within.

You can help yourself by understanding the powers of your mind. Yoga science knows how to control physical pain and has many ways to be free from pain. As far as physical pain is concerned, you may be able to find out its cause and you can help yourself to control that physical pain by your mental powers. But then you find yourself caught by mental pain. As far as mental agony, pain and misery are concerned, you will have to study your desires. You should divide your desires into two parts: those in the outside world and the internal desire to attain happiness. You think that after fulfilling a particular desire, you will be very happy, but later on you find out there are even more desires to be fulfilled. When one desire is fulfilled, another desire creeps in. It seems there is no end in sight.

Philosophy says life is a manuscript you have written, but the beginning and end of the manuscript are missing. Literature says life is a long sentence with many commas and semi-colons but without any full stops; only the middle portion is with you. And still another, life is a tale that has been related by the unknown that keeps going. You should have a powerful aim in life, so that all your little desires can be directed to help you attain that one main desire — to remain happy forever.

According to the sages, the goal of meditation is to be free from all pain and to attain a state called WISDOM. Wisdom is not mere happiness. In life you may be happy for five minutes, and then that happiness is lost. That is not wisdom. WISDOM IS INNER HAPPINESS THAT IS ETERNAL AND CAN NEVER BE LOST, no matter what happens, no matter how much turmoil there is in life. Once you have that wisdom, then the pains and pleasures of the world, these momentary waves in life, will no longer disturb you, because you have known the real value of life.

You identify with the objects of the mind and the world, forgetting that your true nature is peace, happiness and wisdom. Your mind, actions and speech distract you and dissipate your energy so much you cannot maintain that Self-awareness. That is why you are suffering. You often put the blame on the stars or on others. But if you carefully observe your actions, you can help yourself to prevent further problems. First of all, you have to understand that to maintain peace, happiness and wisdom is the purpose of life. To attain the purpose of life, you'll have to find another source of knowledge beyond the level of conventional knowledge that has come through the mind.

When you understand the mystery of life within and without and you understand the nature of the universe, you will have realized the purpose of life. The goal of life is not to be desireless; the GOAL OF LIFE IS TO BE CONSTANTLY AWARE OF THE ABSOLUTE TRUTH. The day that desire comes to you, you will have to direct anything you do, all your speech, thoughts and actions toward that desire. *Desireless* means "not having desires for selfish purposes." You need a powerful desire to meditate and to lead your mind inward to attain Brahman. If you are able to make the whole world a means, you will be there. When all the little waves of the ocean are swallowed by one great wave, that wave becomes very powerful. And so, only one burning desire to know the absolute reality is needed. THE HIGHEST HUMAN DESIRE IS THE DESIRE FOR ENLIGHTENMENT.

SADHANA

Your foremost duty is to practise. All sadhana should be directed toward one goal — to know the Lord of life within. When you become a student of life you realize you need to become an insider so you can systematically fathom the many levels of life and finally go to the center of consciousness. Only then will you understand life as it is.

The charms and temptations of the world are very powerful to attract you. Can you imagine how the power of truth will attract you when you are on the path of truth? Remember, when you start to search for truth, the divine light will guide you. If you are committing a blunder but are following truth you will get help, because truth will guide you. That is the beauty and majesty of truth. The ancient rishis used to cry for a guide because they could not find the way to know the reality. Finally, they realized nothing or no one in the world could guide them. They became so disappointed when no guide was forthcoming that suddenly the light to guide them dawned. When you start to tread the path of light, you too will be guided by that light. If you are lost outside, you become afraid; but if you are lost within yourself, sooner or later you will find what you are looking for.

There are two paths: the path of the external world and the path of the internal world. It is easier to tread the path of the external world than that of the internal world because you have not been trained to do so. Till now, you have been living an isolated life. Neither is it healthy to be introverted nor to behave mechanically in the external world. Patanjali says life in the external world is important, but life within is even more important. You don't need God to understand yourself; you have to be self-reliant and understand yourself independently.

In yoga, sadhana has been divided into two parts — *antaranga* and *bahiranga* — within and without respectively. To create a bridge between the two is the focus of yoga science and philosophy. Through education you get a glimpse of the knowledge of the external world, but nobody teaches you about the world within. Although you may know something about scientific achievements, mind and energy you remain ignorant of how to transform yourself. What you consider to be knowledge cannot help you to transform yourself because that is mere information.

Life in the external world can become disastrous if you don't know how to live. If you were to examine your life in the external world you would probably see a puppet mechanically going through actions. If someone cries, you cry; if someone smiles, you also smile. You may have created a situation for yourself in which you are living with someone you no longer care to live with.

And even though you feel trapped in that situation, you continue to live with it. Perhaps you have bought a house without understanding what is entailed in maintaining a house and now you no longer want to live in that house. Or you may have gone through the process of educating yourself and now you are master in something that is not useful in the world. But you have done it and so you are living with it. You have created many situations like this for yourself that have caused you tension and unhappiness. If you don't like your job yet you keep doing it, this creates conflict in your mind and constant tension within. Wherever there is conflict, there is pain. You have to take interest in what you are doing. If you continue to do something you don't want to do, you are creating more tension and preparing yourself for disease.

The internal path is entirely different. There is a difference between Karma Yoga and Raja Yoga. Karma Yoga helps you to know external life first and then leads you inside, while Raja Yoga says you have to understand samyama and the techniques of concentration, meditation and samadhi. The scriptures explain very little because it's difficult to understand them without the right explanation. It is easy to quote the scriptures, to memorize a few lines from the Vedas, the Upanishads and other scriptures of the yogic tradition, but it is not so easy to live according to yogic science, that which is popularly known as Raja Yoga or Ashtanga Yoga.

Action is definitely inferior to knowledge. Karma leads you to four stages: creation, modification, travel and purification. An example of creation is to make a table out of wood. By modifying milk you can make butter. Third thing, you can go to your destination by travelling. Fourth is purification. Thus, actions can lead you to four stages, but action cannot give you emancipation or liberation. YOU HAVE TO PUT GOLD INTO THE FIRE TO PURIFY IT.

Now, when you are evoking the fire you are doing action (karma). Knowledge is different from action. Tapas is action, but knowledge is not action. However, the tapas of Brahman is knowledge, not action. And knowledge and action are two contrasting ends. Action will give you some result; knowledge from the very beginning has its cause and effect in knowledge. There is no such action that can lead you to Brahman. Actions are performed because human beings cannot live without performing actions. And when you do actions, those actions will bring fruits; and when the fruits come to you they will involve you to do more. It is a continuous chain reaction. To get freedom from this seemingly endless cycle, you should continue to do your actions and offer the fruits of your actions to others.

There are two ways: to know and to practise. People want to know, but they don't want to practise. That is not yoga. Yoga says don't care to know, but care to practise, and then you'll know. Then, you can go to the next step, the royal path. *Satu dirgha kale nirantarya satkara sevito dhridabhumi.* YOU SHOULD PRACTISE EVERY DAY AT THE SAME TIME FOR A LONG TIME WITHOUT ANY BREAK. Patanjali instructed his students to sit every day at the same time so it would become easier to form the habit.

Once I was in search of a quiet place to do sadhana where nobody would disturb me, somebody helped me to find a suitable cave. That cave is called

Sitavani and is near Haldwani, District Nainital. I still visit that place sometimes.

So I sat down, and that man who had helped me to go there, brought some milk, water, tea leaves and sugar. After he had gone, I decided to make tea. But as soon as I would pour the tea into my glass, it would vanish! This happened three times. The third time I became angry. So I thought, *"Bhuta guha."* (*It's a haunted cave!*) *What have I done? I have wasted my time. With disgust I thought, I am trying to do sadhana these days, but instead I am being disturbed by this.*

The fourth time I made tea, three siddhas suddenly appeared. One of them said, "This is our cave; we live here. If you also want to live here, you are most welcome to stay to do your practice. And anything you want, all you have to do is just think of it and it will come."

So, in the morning, I would write out my menu. And what the siddhas had told me was true! Whatever I asked for came! This was very convenient for me. For six months I lived in that cave. But the whole time I was there I could feel there was something wrong in my sadhana.

At the end of six months, I eagerly went to see my master. I bowed as usual and he kicked me. He was very angry. "You always look for the easy way, because we have spoiled you. You searched for a cave where some siddhas were living and now you also have become a great siddha. All you have to do is desire something, and it comes. And you call that sadhana? You should learn the principles of sadhana before you try to do sadhana."

Then he called me many bad names. "Get out of this place and don't come and see me until you have properly completed your sadhana."

A swami may inspire and guide you, but they cannot enlighten you because you are not ready. Therefore, you should do sadhana. Then the day may come when you will be free from all problems and misery. The method for enlightenment has been examined by many sages in the past. Patanjali says this path is fool proof because multitudes have trodden it. This path will lead you to the royal house where the king dwells deep within you in the inner chambers. Here, you will live with the king.

SAMYAMA

NOW, SAMYAMA
SELF-TRANSFORMATION
BENEFITS of SAMYAMA
SANKALPA SHAKTI

NOW, SAMYAMA

Now, you are ready to begin the practice of samyama, which consists of the last three rungs of Ashtanga Yoga — *dharana, dhyana* and *samadhi* (concentration, meditation and samadhi). These three internal techniques will help you to have control over mind and its modifications. In *Vibhuti Pada*, Patanjali describes samyama as the process of inner transformation that leads to enlightenment. *Vibhuti* means "power." Inherent to this state is the acquisition of special powers (siddhis).

Patanjali emphasized you should not postpone enlightenment. You can attain wisdom in this lifetime. To help you do this, he systematized the yogic methods you can use for self-improvement and to attain the higher levels of consciousness. Of these methods, he particularly emphasized the path of samyama (self-transformation), the main topic of *Vibhuti Pada*. One who follows the inner path systematically is on the path of samyama. So far you have been practising the first five rungs of Ashtanga Yoga to deal with external disturbances. These are external methods and include the yamas and niyamas, asana, pranayama and pratyahara. If you have developed the capacity to voluntarily withdraw your mind from the external world, now you have to deal with internal disturbances that are deeper and stronger. Only then can you have perfect control over yourself. Patanjali says there are three internal steps that a student must undertake to understand their internal life. The first five steps have been described in Volume 2 of *Yoga the Sacred Science*. The next three steps are internal in relation to the preceding ones. By combining and integrating these three internal steps you can have control over mind and its modifications.

SAMYAMA is the way to gain deeper knowledge of the qualities or characteristics of an object, and to go to the deeper states of your being where the one consciousness is flowing in various degrees and grades. These three stages are used to understand the various levels of consciousness and are very important in the path of enlightenment. If you do not know the technique of withdrawal of the senses, you cannot have concentration, meditation or samadhi. And concentration is impossible if you do not learn how to pay attention toward the work that you are doing. Likewise, dhyana is not possible without concentration. Finally, if you do not do dhyana, samadhi is not possible.

SELF-TRANSFORMATION

Samyama is a process of inner transformation that takes place in three stages: dharana (concentration), dhyana (meditation) and allowing your mind to flow spontaneously toward the final goal or samadhi. If you want to be courageous and fearless and develop the capacity to fully use your potentials, you will have to attain a higher level of awareness. The differences among the three stages of samyama are as follows: During the practice of dharana you may be remembering your mantra or a sound, you may be focusing on an issue that you have taken up in your mind for the sake of analysis or you may be contemplating a particular idea. Your mind may become distracted for a second or two and go here and there but again it comes back to the point of concentration. This could be concentration, but it is not meditation. If your concentration is not supported by motivation, you may be able to concentrate but you will not understand why you are concentrating. As you progress to the second stage, dhyana, you will come to understand the purpose of concentrating your mind.

Although there are three stages in samyama, they are actually different levels of one process. As you progress through each stage your level of awareness will continue to expand until you reach the most subtle dimensions of your being. By practising samyama you can gain awareness of all the levels of consciousness, including the highest level where you will have freedom from all pain and misery. If you observe a mountain from afar, you cannot see what is behind the mountain. But when you go to the top of the mountain, from there you can see above and below, here, there and everywhere. Similarly, when you go to the source of consciousness and attain the highest state of consciousness you become wise because you see things as they are. Samyama is the way to go safely to the inside world and to understand it. Once you have understood the source of power within you, it will be easy to have peace, happiness and wisdom. By understanding all the levels of consciousness, step by step you can establish inner harmony. Even if it takes a long time, if you persist in the systematic practice of samyama, eventually you will succeed in the process of self-transformation. When you study the internal states of your mind with the help of samyama, you will be able to distinguish between that which is real and that which is not.

If you are convinced that God has created you the way you are, you may think it is not possible to transform yourself. However, once you become aware you are fully responsible for your actions, you definitely can improve and grow. One needs only to have patience, persistence and sincerity to embark on the inner journey that leads to an incomparable treasure within. Patanjali says all human beings can attain the true goal of human life by understanding the aphorisms of the Yoga Sutras and applying them in daily life. In *Vibhuti Pada* he explains that by practising samyama and making your mind one-pointed, you can gradually transform your personality and develop internal awareness of the subtler dimensions of your being and have control over mind and its modifications. In human life the exploration of the external world alone is not considered to be all there is to life. One should learn to understand their internal states so they can better express themself in their external states by such understanding. This transformation results in the settling of distractions and the simultaneous development of one-pointedness that can help you to attain those hidden, unfathomable states of life of which you are not yet aware. Samyama is a way to experiment and study the internal states, gradually fathoming one after another the various levels of consciousness, including the highest level of consciousness.

BENEFITS OF SAMYAMA

Everyone experiences a certain level of awareness, but there are many other levels to attain. Presently, you are aware of only one level of consciousness where you experience pain and joy. No object is absolutely painful or joyful, because all objects have a dual nature. Therefore, nothing can be exclusively painful or joyful. An object that is a source of pain can become a source of joy; likewise, an object that is a source of joy can become a source of pain. For example, you have a new watch that you are enjoying. If it is snatched from you, it will give you pain. So actually, pain and joy have no value in life. If you spend your whole life whining about how painful life is, your mind will remain limited to that level of pain and you will remain unaware there is something higher. Without the practice of samyama you will remain at your current level of consciousness in which suffering consumes your energy.

You need to have a higher level of awareness because you are suffering and that suffering is so painful it is taking all of your energy. Suffering becomes irrelevant once you attain a higher level of awareness and realize that pain and joy are merely relative terms and thus have no true value.

You all are in the bondage you have created for yourself. By thinking you are an individual, you have isolated yourself from the whole. When you isolate yourself from the reality you lose sensitivity toward other human beings. That is why you are suffering from fear, anxiety and pain. You need to expand that individuality to cosmic consciousness. By practising samyama you can understand yourself on all levels and make your mind aware of the highest level of consciousness where you get freedom from pain and misery. When you understand that, you will be able to get rid of pain because you have opened a higher level of awareness from where you will be able to see that all you have now is irrelevant. You will become aware there is something beyond that. When you become aware of the reality, you can never become bitter to anyone. In the state of enlightenment, you just give love. Once you understand the motion of life, then you will float in that joy eternally.

SANKALPA SHAKTI

Sankalpa means "determination." You must have firm determination to change. You want to transform yourself and yet you don't want to make effort. If you sincerely want to transform yourself, first you must build up your sankalpa shakti (firm determination). Determination has three confirmations: I CAN DO IT, I HAVE TO DO IT, AND I WILL DO IT. And once you decide to do something you should not waiver or deviate from that decision. Those who make a confirmation to do something every day but then do not do it are weakening their will power. Many of you don't understand the difference between will power and the will to do something. When mind is fully concentrated, that fully concentrated mind creates will power. The mind is dissipated by the senses. The more you have no control over your mind, the more you do not pay attention toward the things that you do, the more your mind will remain dissipated. The more one-pointed and concentrated the mind becomes, the more dynamic will be your will power. And after you develop will power, you will have self-confidence. Lack of self-confidence is one of the points of failure in your life. When you have self-confidence you can do anything.

Sometimes you may want to do something but you cannot do it or you don't find the means to do it. If you form the habit of wanting to do something but you are not able to do it, you will weaken your will power. You should learn to have strength from the real source of all strength. Will power is essential for self-confidence. One should not be overconfident, but one should not lack confidence. Self-confidence comes after you have observed yourself and watched your capacity. That is the way to build real personal strength.

You cannot imagine how much power you will have when you have a one-pointed mind. When mind remains scattered and is not free, Patanjali prescribes systematic meditation, done with determination. The more will power you have, the more dynamic your personality will be. For that you will have to do a series of exercises on concentration. You should select a particular system or method that helps you to develop concentration. In concentration the scattered, dissipated condition of the mind is trained to become one-pointed. This will lead you to a meditative state. When the mind is concentrated and your will power strengthened, you can have control over your mind and be more fully aware of your capacity. If your mind is one-pointed and inward, then mind can fathom the unknown levels of life. If you follow a system, you will not hallucinate. But if you do it in an unsystematic way, soon you may start to jump or dance, and you might think you are experiencing samadhi or kundalini awakening.

You can get rid of *avidya* (ignorance) by making your mind one-pointed and sharpening your faculty of discrimination so you can discriminate between that which is truth and not truth, that which is eternal and not eternal. For one who is ignorant, they are mingled so deeply it is difficult to separate them. The student should have a very penetrative one-pointed mind like the bees that collect fragrance from many flowers and convert it into honey. This is possible when you start to do meditation.

Rahul Sankrityayan was a great Indian writer who was born in the late nineteenth century in Azamghar. He was also a great explorer, traveler and historian and had written many books even before he became famous. I knew him very well. He was a revolutionary from the very beginning. During those days, landlords under the Indian feudal system used to exploit the peasants who were forced to do labor for them. Because Rahul was opposed to this system one day he sat down and said, "I am not going to eat and I will not move unless you stop taking advantage of poor people."

The landlord was very annoyed by this and decided to release his wild elephant from his stall so he would kill Rahul. This way, nobody would suspect him. However, after having been released, the elephant went near Rahul who was sitting very still, but did nothing to him. He simply turned around and returned to his stall. When the landlord saw what had happened, again he drove the elephant toward that side. He tried three times, but the elephant kept returning. The fourth time the elephant was sent he sat down next to Rahul and put his trunk on his lap. Rahul kissed the elephant.

There are many such stories that are based on fact and the power of determination. With such sankalpa shakti you could do anything. Whatever you do in the external world, you will never receive the results you desire if you do it without determination. If you make a practice schedule for yourself and stick to it, it will not be difficult. By disciplining your thoughts, speech and actions you can completely transform your personality. Even those who say they have given up still want to change. They want to improve themselves and be happy; they want to understand and to know.

Sankalpa shakti is mental power, not physical strength. You have to utilize all the aspects of your mind to support your efforts toward self-transformation. If you want to do something, just do it, no matter what happens. And stop thinking about or doing anything else. In this way you will develop dynamic will and will be able to create wonders in the world. If mind moves, body will also move, but if body moves it is not necessary that mind moves. Many times you force yourself to do things you do not want to do, and if you go on doing this for some time, then your mind will stop moving with your body because you are forcing your body to go against your will. This means you have not understood the relationship of body and mind.

Sankalpa shakti means "will power." In ancient times, the rishis, the great seers always used to remember, *I am this, I am this and I am this. I can do it, I will do it, and I have to do it no matter what happens.* That is sankalpa shakti. Make your mind one-pointed and finally be there.

DHARANA

SUTRA 1: *Desha bandhas cittasya dharana.*

In CONCENTRATION the MIND FLOWS within a LIMITED SPACE and a CERTAIN AREA.

ANTARMUKHA
FULL ATTENTION
ONE-POINTED MIND
the METHOD
FOCAL POINT
CONCENTRATION PRACTICUMS

ANTARMUKHA

According to the first sutra of *Vibhuti Pada,* for concentration you need to keep the mind within a limited area and you have to have an object of concentration on which to focus. In addition, you must have a method to help you focus your mind. Patanjali is talking about concentration within that can lead you to a state of meditation, as opposed to concentration in the external world. Concentration on any external object is not to be confused with dharana. For example, if you concentrate on an object of negativity or worry, that is not dharana. In the external world you can look at an object with a fully concentrated mind, but you cannot know anything merely by concentration. However, you can do things in the external world more accurately if your mind is concentrated. For example, accountants use concentration when they are doing accounting work; a lover is spontaneously concentrated toward their beloved. When you read a book with full concentration that is not the same as the concentration required for meditation. You have learned to concentrate your mind on external things, but you have not learned how to make your mind inwardly one-pointed. You have known something about the external world but you are still a stranger to yourself. To study your internal being, first of all you will have to learn internal concentration or *antarmukha.*

The greatest obstacle in the path of Self-realization is lack of concentration, because it prevents you from seeing things as they are. More importantly, without concentration you cannot do meditation. Many people are afraid to do concentration, because they think it will make them tense, but meditation is not possible without concentration. You cannot watch the capacity of your mind and there is no way to measure your progress if you have not learned how to concentrate. In concentration you consciously allow your mind to flow toward one direction.

FULL ATTENTION

You have all the powers within; you simply need to train yourself. The technique of dharana actually begins with the practice of attention. Attention is the key to success, both within and without. Two things are necessary for you to always be successful in anything you do: how to be still and how to give full attention toward the things that you are doing. If you are trying to concentrate on something, but your mind keeps running away, it means you have not created interest toward that object. There are many reasons why your mind keeps running here and there. You may be hungry or tired or you want to do something else. If your mind is frequently distracted by other thought patterns, it means you have left behind some important things in the unconscious mind. When your mind is preoccupied, it obstructs the remembrance of mantra.

Sometimes you do what you think is the source of your enjoyment, but you do not enjoy being there because your mind is somewhere else. You should learn to enjoy whatever you are doing with both mental and physical coordination. This will happen when you create a real interest for the things that you are doing. All duties — whether they are smaller or larger, higher or more trivial — should be done with interest. If you pay full attention and take interest in anything you do in the external world, you will enjoy what you are doing. Likewise, you won't enjoy any work that you do if you do it half-heartedly without full attention. Most of what you are doing in your daily life, you are doing just for the sake of doing something. You can have powerful concentration if you train yourself.

If you really are sincerely interested in knowing something, the whole secret is not to fight; just allow yourself to know. You need to create genuine interest in order to know the things that are before you. Why do people think about something before they do it? Because doing itself is not very important; the enjoyment is not in the action. When you do an action it is only an expression of enjoyment. Learn to enjoy things by putting your whole heart and mind into them, and then you will really enjoy them. THE REAL ENJOYMENT LIES IN YOUR MIND AND HEART ALONE.

If you act based on what you think and pay attention to your thoughts and actions, you will be preparing yourself for the practice of dharana. By paying attention to your actions in the external world, you are slowly training your mind. The more you pay attention, the more aware you become. As you increase your awareness of those things you are doing that you know you should not do, you will no longer enjoy doing them. It is important to keep your mind with your actions instead of allowing yourself to do anything automatically. Automatic does not mean you are doing something without any cause; everything has a cause. If you pay more attention toward the things that you do, not only will you strengthen your mind, mind will also slowly become one-pointed. Sometimes attention is conscious, and sometimes it becomes unconscious. For example, you unconsciously look after your child more and more when you love your child. There is something inside you that inspires you to pay attention toward your child.

Attention is not possible without interest. If you do not create interest in the duties you are performing or in the practices you are doing, mere repetition is not going to help you. The obstacles will be there and it will be difficult to remove them. You cannot establish yourself in your real nature if your mind doesn't agree to go forward because it's afraid to do something more. Any time you do something you don't want to do you weaken your will power. If you want to do something, do it! And don't say you have committed a mistake. If you are killed, if you are hit or if you are jailed, then that is your responsibility. When you do something, know that you are doing it and accept the responsibility for the consequences. In this way, your will power is not weakened and you can learn from society what is right and what is wrong. If you are doing wrong, society will kick you. You never should complain that you have committed a mistake and you are sorry. You say sorry 100 times to acknowledge your mistake. That will create a complex in your heart and mind. Nothing should influence you, impress you or affect you. If you allow the external world to toss you around, you cannot be guided by the Self within. You have to be very strong from within.

Without the ability to concentrate, you will never be able to meditate. At best you will be able to create a state of nothingness in which you lose touch with both the unconscious and conscious mind. When you pay attention and take interest in your duties there will be no tension. By paying attention you are making your mind one-pointed and inward. Once mind is made inward, the next step is concentration. Concentration should lead you inwardly to a one-pointed mind, not outwardly. Then, concentration will flow into meditation without any interruption and that will strengthen your practice. At times you may come back to physical consciousness, at other times you will go ahead.

ONE-POINTED MIND

After learning to turn the mind inward, you have to make your mind one-pointed. Attention requires a one-pointed mind. The mind of the beginning student has the habit of flowing outward and becoming dissipated in the external world. You will have to make constant effort to turn the mind inward. It will take time to form this habit, and it can create problems in your worldly life at first, because the mind is storing a reservoir of thoughts, ideas, symbols, fancies and fantasies in the unconscious.

Life should not be ruled by don'ts, restrictions or limitations. There should be some understanding of knowledge and inner strength. If you continue to give the step-by-step method to mind, it will not run. In meditation you are asking the mind to become inward and one-pointed. For this, first you have to work with your body. When you are done with the body, you have won one-fourth the battle. With a one-pointed mind, whether external or internal, your perception will be clearer. For example, when you are reading, you understand and retain what you are reading only if your mind is concentrated. The dissipated mind cannot remember what has been read. You cannot retain what you are studying if your mind is somewhere else. I was told not to study when my mind is not cooperating. The mind plays very subtle tricks. If you are lazy, mind will encourage you to go to sleep by convincing you to postpone your work for tomorrow or day after tomorrow. Then, you will go on postponing for tomorrow. If you concentrate when you are reading something you will remember what you have read. When you read you should retain what you are reading and be able to recall it later. When you know something you know it and when you want to recall it you should easily be able to because you have known it before. When you concentrate, you should try to become aware of your unconscious mind. Even though you don't want to remember, worry or be involved with what is coming from the unconscious, more and more thoughts come. This is natural.

For truly understanding any object in the world you need a one-pointed mind. Only a pure mind can attain one-pointedness. When you are not attentive, you hear only a small part of what is being said, and then you say you don't understand. Or if you are fanatic and rigid in your views and are not open to understanding, the same thing will happen. There are two types of one-pointedness. Mind can become negatively one-pointed if you keep brooding on the same thing: *I am going to die, I am bad, I am ill.* If you give such negative feedback to yourself and repeatedly condemn yourself, there is no remedy in the world that will help you. Self-condemnation leads to sickness and loss of self-confidence. Remember that you belong to God and you have no right to condemn that which is not yours. Forgive yourself for the mistakes you have committed.

You tend to label a person as good or bad, instead of taking the time to study that person as a subject. When you go to a psychiatrist they never judge you as being good or bad. They study you as you are from your behavior, expressions and emotions. You also should study yourself without making any judgment. It hardly comes in your mind that you are a good person because you need someone to tell you that you look beautiful, you are wonderful and you are a very good person. If you are not told that, then you do not realize your good qualities. And if ten people come to you again and again and say there is something wrong with you, I assure you the next day you are going to visit a psychiatrist.

Society has taught you this feeling of self-condemnation. You allow other people to make you feel that you are bad, you are very small and you are not powerful. And so, you forget that you are powerful. This you have learned unconsciously from the environment. Unconscious teaching is more powerful than conscious teaching. Consciously or unconsciously your mind has to be trained in concentration. If it is not concentrated, meditation is not possible. Outward concentration will not lead you to a state of meditation. Your concentration should be turned inward, not outward. If that is too difficult for you, to begin with you can concentrate your mind on an external object. For example, you can light a lamp and gaze at the flame. That is *trataka*. This is the way to train the eyes, but it is not meditation. It may help you to concentrate better so you can become a better accountant, dancer or musician. When you light a lamp or light, the first color you find is black because the light is not full. Then immediately a fierce color comes. Those who have accomplished the practice of external concentration to make their mind one-pointed by concentrating on the burning flame of a candle can see the whole range of colors.

THE METHOD

Mind has the capacity to export and import both. What you export is your choice; but you don't know how to select what your mind imports and you don't know how to handle that random input. You think the objects of the world force themselves into your mind, but that never happens. Sometimes you even try to push this responsibility onto God. You have to understand you are doing it yourself. Your mind receives incoming impressions based on your interests. In this way your mind becomes a source of problems for you, but you can also make it a means of liberation if you understand the method of how to make your mind inward. The important concept to remember here is YOUR LIBERATION IS IN YOUR HANDS.

For inward concentration, there is a particular method:

• First, see that your body does not move, yet it is steady and comfortable.
• Next, your breath should be calm and serene and you should be completely relaxed.
• Third, mind goes on with its thinking process, yet you are not disturbed.
• Fourth, if you have a focal point or a mantra you should understand what it is and how to use it.

FOCAL POINT

To begin the practice of concentration, it is easier to concentrate the mind on some object or image, because the mind has a natural tendency to visualize and go outward. This object of concentration or meditation is a difficult task. Some temperaments are not capable of concentrating on subtle objects. One must have something to tie the mind to such as a theme, word, light or other object. The sages had explained that to focus the mind there must be something else — either a word or a symbol — that is the projection of an idea. When you have a focal point, then your mind will come back from here, there and everywhere and will be concentrated on that automatically. Without a focal point, mind will continue to roam around. The object of concentration should not be the body, which is subject to change, death, and decay, nor the breath or mind. There are already so many objects and symbols in your mind, so many ideas, fancies and fantasies, it will not help you to add one more. Today you meditate on an object, and tomorrow you find you have added another impression to the already millions of impressions in your mind. That is not concentration. The purpose of having an object of concentration is to consciously strengthen that particular object so that whenever you want to disperse all the impressions of your mind and remain with that object, it can be helpful to you. If you cannot do that, you are just creating another ripple in the ocean in which there are already millions of ripples.

If you want to increase your capacity for concentration you can choose a particular color or light, but that is not meditation. If you have an object to focus on during concentration, after some time your concentration will be strengthened till it becomes meditation. And once that flow swallows all other desires, it becomes deep meditation. You may decide to make the inner light your object of concentration. Intellectually, this sounds very good, but it is not easy to concentrate upon something that is so abstract. There are other objects that are pleasing and at the same time help the mind to be concentrated. We will discuss mantra as an object of concentration in the next section.

CONCENTRATION PRACTICUMS

CONCENTRATION PRACTICUM 1:

In a comfortable seated position with your eyes closed, you should slowly mentally travel down the body to locate muscle tension while trying to determine from where that tension is coming. From the top of your head go down to your toes and come back. Then repeat. One foot apart from you and exactly before you, mentally visualize a candle with a white base and a blue light that is burning. You are exhaling exactly to the candlelight and inhaling from your candlelight to the crown of your head. If you cannot imagine a blue light, don't worry. You may hear very subtle sound vibrations coming from within. Just listen to them. Exhale and inhale again. Go to the candlelight mentally and come back again to the crown of your head by inhaling, and without any retention, mentally exhale to the candlelight. When you have completely inhaled you should start to visualize the letters of the alphabet from A to Z, allowing the breathing to continue. Having completed the visualization of the alphabet, again consciously inhale and exhale smoothly. Now visualize A to Z only on the space between the two eyebrows. Then, again pay attention to your breath, inhaling and exhaling slowly. Now, ask your mind to listen to the sound vibrations coming from your pineal gland center, then again inhale and exhale deeply. Gently open your eyes.

CONCENTRATION PRACTICUM 2:

The following exercise of visualization is very helpful for enhancing the memory and for making a distracted mind more focused. This exercise can also be used to improve your eyesight. You can best use your mind for even the smallest enjoyment if mind is one-pointed. Whatever you do, your mind should be there. It's the nature of mind to attend to one thing at a time. Just watch how many times your mind slips from this train of drawing A-Z. When mind is distracted it means you are doing something but thinking of something different.

Keep the eyes open and keep the mind with the movement of the eyes as you mentally draw each alphabet. I have drawn A first, now I have drawn B. I am drawing E now. If you train a child to do this exercise, you will find that child will become immensely powerful.

Initially, you can do it with the eyes open; but when you're actually doing this practice you should close your eyes. If you hook up to an EEG and you make your eyes still, there should be no movement. You should have control over even the movement of your eyes.

When you can draw all the lines of the letters without any break, you have done concentration. What initially happens is that your mind will slip and forget to draw a letter. This means your mind is not organized. This has also proved to be very helpful for loss of memory and absentmindedness.

You should visualize the letters very large so your eyes are moving a good deal. Large letters are always good. I have practised it in Urdu also, and in Persian. I was able to easily memorize all the letters of these alphabets by doing this practice. There is a method for learning language by sound, not by grammar. With this method you can learn any language in 18 days' time, provided you use your memory properly.

CONCENTRATION PRACTICUM 3:

You can expand your conscious mind through the following practice of concentration. First day, close your eyes and remember the number one. What usually happens is that instead of remembering the number one, different numbers will keep coming. But if you keep trying, after a few days you will find that you can hold it for a few seconds. If you continue to practise, gradually the amount of time it holds your attention will increase. In this way you can slowly expand the conscious mind and stop the external flow of the mind. You can choose any external point for concentration. For the first few days you will want to concentrate on something that is pleasing to the mind, such as your girlfriend's photograph or image, or on certain thought forms. After a short time that image will disappear and many distractions will come to your attention. So, there are two difficulties: Mind does not want to remain on something unpleasant; and if the object is pleasant, it can lead to many distractions.

the Science of Mantra

SOUND, VIBRATIONS AND SYMBOLS

Now, I'm explaining to you the relationship between sound and form. How sound is related to form is a science. Every sound produces a pattern and its corresponding form, because form and sound are intermingled. This whole material world was produced from sound, but only God knows what that sound was. The Bible says, "In the beginning was the word, and the word was God." Many sages have tried to interpret this, but God alone knows which sound manifested the world.

Likewise, all human beings have manifested from sound. The science of mantra explains it. If I give you a mantra, the vibrations of that mantra create a form that is working for you, even though you don't know it. Many times you are doing something you should not do, and immediately that form will stop you. For example, you may want to do a business that would not be successful. That form will create something to prevent you from doing it. Or, you are about to have an accident because you are driving recklessly. If you have created that sound so strongly that it has really become a form, that form can even stop you from having an accident.

You should be aware that every spoken word has been preceded by a thought. This implies the basis of communication is not words but thoughts, because a thought is virtually a word or group of words. When a thought travels it creates a sound, and when sound travels it vibrates and produces a symbol. The vibrations create patterns that are actually symbols of the thought. If you take a slate and spread some fine powder over it, and blow a sound from here, the vibrations of the sound will travel to the slate and will create a certain pattern in the powder. In this way, SOUND CAN LEAD YOU TO A PARTICULAR IMAGE.

When I was studying homeopathy at Hamburg University people used to approach me because they had heard I was a young swami who had come from a great tradition and that my guru was great. They asked me if there was any way to do experiments to find out if you create the sound OM, would it make a pattern as seen in the books. I told them to first draw all the possible patterns they had seen. Then, we chose an ancient one. In order to continue our experiment, I asked them to bring the most ancient musical instrument, the conch shell. When they brought it they did not know how to blow it, so I blew it and it made the sound, *OMMMMMMM*. Having made a big board, we blew from every corner and it always drew out the symbol of OM.

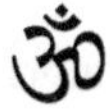

In the Book of Revelations John describes experiences of sounds combined with visions. If you sit quietly, you will notice in your thinking process two things: An image comes, followed by another image, and between the two images there is a gap. So sound and images are very closely related. When John would hear the sound of a drum he would turn his eyes and he would have a vision. And whenever he would see that same vision again, he would also hear the sound of the drum. So, the sound brought about the vision and vice versa. In this way the sound and image led him to the deeper levels of his being. This was during the period when Christianity was under persecution, and he was very worried that the message of Jesus Christ would not be spread far and wide because many priests and teachers were being persecuted. He was so concentrated during those days he started to have visions of the flame of love.

No matter which form you use—Christ on the cross, Christ as a little baby, Christ as a very healthy, handsome man who turned water into wine or Christ who blesses everyone—they are all symbols. I do not worship those that are called gods in Hinduism because they are symbols. The symbol of the cross is prominent in Christianity. The cross represents the two hemispheres of the body, upper and lower. Christians do not understand the symbol of the cross. A necktie is actually symbolic of a cross. Christ died on the cross for the sake of selfless service. It has come into fashion to wear a necktie. If you do not wear a tie and go to your office, you are not considered to be well dressed. But the actual meaning of the necktie is to remember Christ all the time. The cross also represents the internal states of human beings. There are three chakras above, three chakras below, and in the center is the Sacred Heart. The flames of your efforts go up, the blessings come down.

There are cultures that have a very profound science of symbolism. Every sound has a form, and every form can be used. You always think in symbols in your mind. Many times you cannot interpret your own symbols or dreams because you don't study the symbols that your thoughts create. Symbols actually make up a different language. As you study body language and breathing habits you will have to study the symbols of your mind. Before you can study them properly you will have to first put them into categories. But you should not do this while you are meditating, because otherwise you will be spending all your time thinking and categorizing your thoughts.

MANTRA DEFINED

You should understand the science of mantra and how mantra's vibrations help your entire being. Mantras are unstruck sounds *(anahata nada)* that flow from the center of silence within. Clapping the hands is a struck sound; unstruck sounds were originally experienced by the ancient sages in a deep state of meditation in that vast silence within. Though gentle but powerful, those sacred sounds were captivating and joyful. They are called mantras or *bijas* (seeds). The word *mantra* comes from its Sanskrit root, *mananat trayate iti,* which means "that which dispels the darkness of ignorance, pain and misery." Beneath all your thoughts you have to maintain constant awareness of the center of reality within. A mantra can help you to maintain that center of awareness.

A mantra is a set of sacred sounds or syllables imparted by a competent teacher to be used as an object of concentration. Mantra helps your mind to become one-pointed and that's all. There is no need to go beyond that or try to find out the various meanings and applications of mantra. If you observe yourself you will see that when you want to concentrate on something, your mind runs away. You can easily watch how many times your mind flies away from your mantra. This means you have not created any interest toward the object on which you want to concentrate. If you are not motivated to do the practice of concentration then you are merely going through the motions of concentrating without understanding why you are doing it. You should convince yourself to do these practices by studying sacred books, listening to your teacher and becoming familiar with the wisdom of the sages. For the sutras, you need a teacher to give you an explanation; for mantra, once you have it, you do not need any guidance, because mantra will guide itself. Mantra helps to purify the mind of pain and misery. As a representative of the Lord, mantra can help you to reach samadhi. Mantra and meditation go hand in hand. Meditation is a process and mantra is a tool that creates a bridge, *pranava setu,* for going from this side of life to the unknown.

There are various types of mantra, but there is nothing like inferior or superior mantra. All religious and spiritual traditions of the world know how powerful the great sayings are that the sages imparted to their disciples and they all have some sort of mantra or sacred word they remember. In all the great traditions you will find different types of mantras. They are all valid and their meaning is one and the same. Each type is to be repeated in a specific manner and each has a different effect. It is not necessary that you have a Hindu mantra; it could be a Jewish mantra. You may have seen Jewish people reading their small book, or you have probably seen Christians remembering a prayer to Mother Mary with their rosary beads. They are remembering "Hail Mary, Hail Mary, Hail Mary." By repeating this prayer they are unconsciously strengthening the form of Mother Mary.

The mantras for meditation are in a different category. They do not create obstacles to your breathing process and are easy for the mind, ultimately leading the mind to the silence. You can meditate without a mantra also, but then you will have to experiment and be your own judge. You might fail or by chance you could gain.

There is a vast difference between mantra and ordinary language. Whereas words are known by their meaning, mantras and bijas are known by their particular vibrations. It is very interesting to study how sound vibrations affect you. Mantra is a soothing sound that vibrates, strengthens and relaxes your nervous system. It is not a religious word and has nothing to do with any religion. Mantra contains the entire philosophy of life. This is true in yoga, all darshanas and all the religious scriptures in the world. You don't have to study books or search anywhere if you really understand your mantra and you rely on it and work with it. However, if you speak the mantra out loud, the sound vibrations will dissipate and be wasted. If you speak a mantra outside, it becomes gross but if you remember it mentally it has a very subtle effect. Ordinary words and sounds are dissipated in the external world, but the vibrations of the mantra will lead you deeper and deeper within, to the vibrant silence and calmness from where we have all come.

TEACHER'S ROLE

Patanjali says you should gradually progress from the gross to the subtle, then to the subtler and finally to the subtlest level of consciousness. Before a child is born the embryo develops through many different forms. Likewise, when you are growing spiritually, your personality goes through many changes. You have to be very vigilant in order to observe those transformations. Up to a certain point, the student of yoga can prepare themself, but beyond that point guidance is required. A teacher who guides as part of a lineage or legitimate tradition can help a student to systematically advance. This may take place in a series of important steps, the first of which is the students' initiation in which they receive a mantra on which to concentrate. You need to have an object on which mind can focus such as a mantra, but the object should not make your mind pensive or introverted. Teachers impart mantras to prepared students to help focus the mind in the practice of meditation. Many people come for initiation, but sometimes I suddenly feel I should not initiate a certain person, so I tell them to come another day. When they come again, I might tell them I'm busy. I torture them like this because I want to know how determined they are. If I make the effort to till the land and impart a seed to you, it is up to you to sow it. If you are lazy and don't want to work then you think the teacher has not done anything. A teacher should do everything for the students and should not expect anything from them, or else the students will always disappoint the teacher. I don't expect anything from you and so I am never disappointed. Expectation is the mother of all problems. When the student comes to a teacher, they come with many expectations because they think the teacher will give everything. The teacher gives 50%, but the other 50% is your own work. No matter how much you try to please me, I will never be pleased. And however much you try to annoy me, I will never become annoyed. I am simply doing my duty toward you and I want to see you happy.

You should honor and serve your teacher with humility and learn from them how to control your mind. If you have a flame for learning you will have a love for your teacher. The more intense is your burning flame for knowledge, the more will be your love for your teacher. If you don't have a flame for learning and you give some fruits to your teacher, then next day some flowers and third day some dollars, it indicates the flame is dying out. I want to see the flame in you but I am only seeing fruits, flowers and dollars. It is the flame that will please the teacher. The other things are secondary and are just friendly formalities. A friend is different from a teacher. A TEACHER IS A DIVINE FRIEND. A mere friend is selfish. If you give them a cup of tea, they will expect two cups from you. The teacher gives you everything, and never expects anything in return. The student tortures the teacher and gives them pain and many such things, but the teacher is accustomed to it. LOVE FOR KNOWLEDGE IS THE ONLY WAY TO PLEASE A TEACHER.

By observing the student, the teacher can know if they are ready to get a particular practice. The moment the student walks in, the teacher should know what type of student they are and for what purpose they need a mantra. If the teacher is experienced, they cannot be cheated. The teacher observes the gestures the student makes, the way they talk, their behavior and their way of writing, reading or understanding. Then the teacher recommends a particular systematic method according to the student's ability and capacity. The teacher immediately concentrates their mind to find the prime problem of the student and then they give the mantra that will help the student. There are some people who intellectualize too much. On the other hand, there are some who are very active, while others are more emotional. In this way an accurate prescription is given to the student according to their characteristics, just as a doctor gives medicine to a patient. The teacher imparts the mantra and asks the student to repeat it and remember it. They then explain the vibrations of the seed they are giving. After some time your mind will naturally follow the mantra. In the preliminary steps you can use a *mala* (a string of beads) to repeat the mantra. Adjusting the mantra with your breath and remembering it all the time are also preliminary.

REMEMBERING MANTRA

In I.28 sutra Patanjali has explained: *Taj japas tad artha bhavanam.* By meditating on the meaning of the mantra, you can attain the highest state. To remember the mantra and to meditate on the meaning of the mantra are two different things. There is a subtle difference between these two words. If you merely remember the mantra, it is not going to help you. It is important to remember the sound constantly so you can watch the capacity of your mind.

When I stayed with Gandhiji in my youth, he would talk about *ajapa japa* and how to remember mantra. *Japa* means "remembrance," *ajapa* means "remembering yet not remembering." The mantra is coming on its own because it has become an unconscious habit and part of your life. You no longer have to make a conscious effort to remember your mantra for it has become part of your life and you spontaneously remember it. This is ajapa japa—to remember your mantra without effort. When the unconscious mind assimilates mantra, then ajapa japa starts. When mantra becomes part of your life, it becomes the predominant habit of the mind in the unconscious that is the reservoir of all your thought patterns.

You can deal with the conscious mind if you develop unconscious activity through the practice of japa. Patanjali says japa should not be done superficially and mechanically. Either you will be remembering your mantra unconsciously or you will be aware of the reality within yourself. Then, the conscious functioning of mind will not affect you. Your unconscious mind remains in a state of tranquillity when you are aware of the reality. You are living here, yet you are there. How much are you here and how much are you there? Some people are here two-thirds of the time and the rest there; others are there most of the time and here only one-fourth of the time. Slowly you can progress until you finally reach the highest state where actually you are here and there simultaneously. No matter where you are or what you are doing, you should develop the habit that you are all the time conscious of your mantra or the reality. Japa will immediately help you to control disorganized emotions. Constant remembrance of mantra is the greatest of all wisdom. I am talking about mantra meditation in which the time comes when mind starts to follow mantra so that mantra and manas become one. Now, if you have doubt that it might happen or it might not happen, then there is only a small chance it will happen. It's very important to remember the mantra without any doubt and with firm faith. Then, mantra will finally take you to the silence or to fulfill your desires.

If you do japa technically in the beginning, after some time you will find trust in your mantra and great joy. No matter how silently you remember your mantra, the tongue will move a little bit. Japa is something you speak. Whenever you are doing japa and remembering your mantra, thoughts will keep coming. If you do japa continuously and nothing intervenes, that is meditation. When you practise meditation, you live in the world and yet remain above.

MANTRA AS FRIEND

When you start to remember your mantra, you will understand that for some time it will be difficult. Initially, you may also find that you are remembering it technically without feeling anything. Sometimes you forget, then again you remember. You say you keep remembering your mantra but nothing is happening, so there must be something wrong somewhere. Even if you are doing it half-heartedly, it will have an effect, because the japa you do is stored in the reservoir of your unconscious mind. It will help you during trying times when there is no one else to help you. A time will come when you will be all alone on this journey. In this time of dire need, when you are all alone and no one can help you to take the voyage from the known to the unknown, mantra will lead you. The best use of remembering your mantra is to be a friend to you when you are leaving this world. That's why the Upanishads say mantra is a bridge from this shore to the other shore, from the known to the unknown. When body, breath and conscious mind fail, your mantra will come forward. At the time of transition, you will not be able to speak or communicate with anyone—not your doctor, your friends, your wife or husband, your children or other people who are dear to you. You cannot take your family, friends or possessions with you while you are in the process of leaving the body and you will feel very lonely. At that time your tongue cannot move, your eyes want to see but there is a haze over everything as darkness creeps upon you and takes over. As consciousness starts to fail, the eyes will no longer have sight; you will want to speak, but you can no longer communicate. You may have millions of dollars in the bank, all your friends are at your disposal, and the doctor is there, but no one can help you. When no one else can help you, that japa will come forward to help you. Therefore, you should not feel that you are not gaining anything in meditation. If you have created a very strong groove in your unconscious by strengthening your mantra over a long time, when you are leaving this world, mantra will come forward and will be your friend. You will need this friend to guide you because many latent thoughts and all the merits and demerits of your life that you have stored in the unconscious will come forward and disturb you. That's why you should always try to have good thoughts. You have to prepare for that day. If you learn how to not involve yourself with the objects of the world, then that transition from life to death will become easy.

As long as your mantra is with you, you are not alone. Who makes you lonely? Your friends and your family whom you love and respect make you lonely. If your husband does not come on time or does not pay attention to you, you become lonely. You will remain lonely as long as you depend on external crutches. Once you become aware of the friend within, you will never feel lonely. You should have a companion who will be there to help you when nobody else can help. If you need money, food or water, your friends can help you. But if you are worried, nobody can share your mental anxiety. Who will help you during that period? If you don't have a companion where will you go? You will become emotionally upset. If you start the process of self-therapy you will gradually fathom all the levels within.

I have so much faith in my mantra, even if you were to tell me you were going to put me in the fire just now, I would not be disturbed. You should have your mantra with you all the time. Let mantra become your constant friend and companion. Because my mantra is my friend and is with me all the time, I am never lonely. You have to be one with your mantra. When mantra itself exists and you no more exist, then mantra can work through you. And if you decide to make it your friend, mantra will always guide you and lead you to the subtler aspects of your being and to the silence within. Silence does not lie within the domain of your mind; SILENCE LIES BEYOND YOUR MIND. Mantras vibrate within when they are silently remembered, so the student is taught to silently meditate on the mantra. But it is not sufficient to just remember the mantra. Through the mantra you can develop awareness of the reality. Because mantra has come from the silence, it has the power to lead you back to the silence, or to the fourth state of turiya.

MEANING OF MANTRA

You should understand the meaning of your mantra and the vibrations of your mantra, and remember it. Even in the beginning, if you don't have faith you should still remember it. If you do something, you are bound to reap the fruits. If you take poison without faith, even then it will affect you.

When I visited a monastery in Tibet, the lamas kept repeating, OM MANI PADME HUM, OM MANI PADME HUM, OM MANI PADME HUM. I asked one of them why they were doing this and he said, "It's a secret. You are not initiated so we cannot tell you the secret." They were worshiping a book that had been written on handmade paper. That book was covered with a thick layer of sandalwood paste. The head priest had told them that anybody who tried to read it would become blind. So, of course nobody would dare attempt to read it. I became very excited because I was always looking for such things. I thought, *Now, I have come to the right place. If I get blind after reading it, it is all the better! I am already blind because I know nothing.* That night I sneaked back to that book. I had a little flashlight with me and I opened the book. I could not read many pages because there was so much sandalwood paste. I found out it was a book of Sanskrit grammar. The lamas did not know what it was and they were worshiping it. The teacher did not know how to explain what was in the book so he told the students to just worship it. And so, they had been worshipping it since ages, without knowing what it was they were worshipping.

NAMAHA

Most mantras that are given in initiation have at the end the word *namaha*. *Namaha* means "nothing belongs to me; everything belongs to Thee." Though you are constantly remembering that nothing belongs to you, the next moment you say, "No, no, no! That is mine." That will certainly create a conflict in your mind. Okay, from the worldly viewpoint, you can say, "This is my partner, this is my house." Yet you are not supposed to be attached to the things of the world because attachment creates misery. When you are constantly remembering, *Oh Lord, nothing belongs to me,* you are remembering yourself and the Lord and the relationship between the Lord and yourself. *All the things I have are yours; nothing belongs to me. I am grateful to you for having given all of this to me.* The entire philosophy of self-surrender is in this mantra.

In Sanskrit *namaha* also means *"namaskara."* Wishing others with folded hands means "I pray to the Brahman in you." This is not a gesture for a human being; it's a gesture for the Brahman that you see in others. When you use this gesture, you cannot fight with anyone, you cannot hate anyone and you cannot injure, hurt or kill anyone. When you say *namaskara* and place the hands together in prayer position at the center of the chest you are saying, "I acknowledge the Lord of life in you." This is where the soul and the Lord meet, and that is the aim of life. So you are not bowing in front of the human being, but to the Lord of life who is within every person. Similarly, when you visit somebody, you should understand you are not just visiting a physical person, but the Lord of the life force that dwells within that person. Your prayer should be so intense that you become one with Brahman and you are lost in Brahman consciousness.

BHAVA AND FEELING

Bhava (feeling) comes later on. Once you fully understand the meaning of your mantra, you will start to recognize the feeling of it. And when you start to feel it, you need to strengthen that feeling. Once that feeling is strengthened, you will no longer be simply remembering the mantra; you will be there because you are remembering it with bhava. Bhava is different from *vichara* (thought) and finer than form. *Bhava* means "that which has come from emotion." In other words, bhava is your emotional body. That emotional body in the lake of mind is constantly being agitated by external stimuli, because the world is full of charms, temptations and attractions that distract your mind. The emotional body can disturb the whole lake because it is so powerful! You don't have to force it because it is already there. However, you have to make human effort and know how to use your mantra. If you sit back and wait your whole life for bhava to come, thinking that God is great, it will never come. You cannot enjoy that bhava, which is definitely superior to all other charms, unless you make sincere efforts. To create bhava you need to encounter your mantra and understand the relationship between mind and mantra. Then your mantra will become bhava, and bhava will become your mantra. Mantra should be repeated with feeling and meaning. When you practice mental repetition of your mantra for a long time, it becomes a part of your nature and you enjoy it. You should remember your mantra so much that it permeates your unconscious and flows spontaneously so you can always remain aware of the reality. Wherever you go and when you are quiet, let your mantra turn into feeling, and LET THAT FEELING BECOME A WAVE OF BLISS WITHIN YOU.

HOW TO USE MANTRA

How to use mantra is a great skill. Mantra works through a particular chakra. For example, if you use a mantra by meditating at muladhara, the base chakra, its effect will be different than if you meditate on any of the other chakras. If you use the same mantra while concentrating on your manipura chakra, it will have a different effect. And if you remember that same mantra on the space between the two eyebrows, the effect will again be totally different. If you remember your mantra all the time, without concentrating on any chakra, the effect also will be completely different. What I have found out, those words or sounds that are considered to be mantras, if they are imparted with love by someone who knows the science, and if they are taken by someone who sincerely wants to practise, they can do tremendous good both in worldly prosperity and in spiritual enlightenment.

CONCENTRATION AND THE CHAKRAS

It is not good for you to choose a chakra center yourself. You should let your teacher guide you. When you get a mantra, you should ask your teacher to give you the point on which mind should be focused. A competent teacher understands at what level of energy your mind dwells, so they can recommend to you a chakra center on which you can focus your mind. This is a science in itself. It becomes a practical science when you learn to use mantra with concentration on a particular chakra. If you are physically unwell, then the navel center (manipura chakra or the solar plexus) should be your meditation focal point. To those who are emotional, the teacher gives anahata chakra as the focal point; and to those who are intellectual, they give ajna chakra. These are the three most profound centers the teacher gives to the student.

MANIPURA CHAKRA AND SOLAR SCIENCE: The teacher gives first a sound and then a mantra to anyone who suffers on account of bad digestion. This sound activates and brings forward the power of the solar system. This is solar science. The solar system is a very complex network of energy patterns in the body that is located at manipura chakra, the navel center. That complex network is called the *kanda* in yogic literature. Those who have a problem with digestion or who have sexual problems are asked to focus on the kanda to activate it. If you come in touch with the solar system or solar power you'll be able to attain good health.

ANAHATA CHAKRA: If your nature is emotionally predominant then you can concentrate on the heart center (anahata chakra), the space between the two breasts. Anahata chakra divides the upper hemisphere from the lower and helps to guide emotional power to emotional maturity. Here two triangles meet to form a six-pointed star. One triangle flows downward, and the other flows upward. The upward flowing triangle represents the ascending force; and the downward flowing triangle is the descending force. The ascending force comes from human effort. If you sincerely make all the effort you can, that can be termed as the ascending force. The descending force is grace.

Your emotional life seems to never be at rest as it is constantly tossed by your thought patterns. You have cultured your mind by education, but you do not know how to culture your emotional life. Because society does not allow wild behavior, there is a tendency to bottle up emotions such as anger, jealousy and greed. You have to behave properly and express your emotions as accepted by society. If you know how to work with your emotions and can control them you can use them as a great power for creativity. But they can also make you sick and destroy you.

If you examine your emotions you will find they all have something to do with something external. Emotions exist because you have established a relationship with some object in the external world that is related to your desires for food, sex, sleep or self-preservation and you suffer because of that. Although you have allowed your mind to become full of negative emotions, you have to realize that is not your true nature. The way to train the emotions is to allow them to go through the thinking process. If you cannot control your emotions, you will have to control your mind. You have to be calm to study yourself on all levels. Once you know how to calm down your mind, you can see anything that is going on there, for mind is a mirror. To calm down the mind you need meditation. That which your emotional life tells you to do in the external world, you can do the same thing during meditation or in your dreams.

Emotion, which is more powerful than the thinking process, can also become a right source of knowledge if you know and understand how to direct that power that can lead you to the height of ecstasy in a second's time. Many great sages have attained the height of wisdom and knowledge because they had reached the height of ecstasy. There, mind does not intervene and cannot reason why this has happened.

A good human being is one who has learned how to integrate a sound mind, a healthy body and a good heart. You need to understand the integration of body, mind and heart. When you try to analyze something intellectually, you have to put your emotions aside. Up to now you have not understood anything about emotions. You often say emotions make you blind, but that is not true. You cannot depend on the intellect because it gathers data from the external world, which is subject to change, death and decay. The data that is gathered by the intellect has not been purified and has no support of the other faculties of mind. Therefore, such data collection does not help you. By contemplating and concentrating on anahata chakra, you can have control over your emotions and thus experience perfect equilibrium and tranquillity.

VISHUDDHA CHAKRA: If you are an artist or a dancer, or if you are creatively inclined, the hollow of the throat (vishuddha chakra) is where you should concentrate.

AJNA CHAKRA: If you are intellectual and always want to reason or intellectualize, then the space between the two eyebrows (ajna chakra) should be your focus. Those who are prepared are asked to meditate at ajna chakra, the gateway to the city of life. *A* means "little," *jna* means "knowledge." You can gain a little knowledge when you meditate on this chakra. According to the scriptures, so far you have not obtained real knowledge because your knowledge is only partial. You will experience real knowledge only when you focus your mind on the space between the two eyebrows. There is a tiny circle on the space between the two eyebrows and on both sides of the circle there is one petal. The two petals of the symbol of ajna chakra are representative of your two eyes. But now you'll see that there are many geometrical figures: the square, triangle and the circle. All other figures are modifications of these three shapes; there cannot be a fourth. The difficulty comes because mind does not want to stay inside a circle but prefers triangles and squares. In the center of the circle there is an unflinching flame steadily burning like a milky, white light. This center is called ajna chakra or *divya chakshu,* the third eye. By concentrating and focusing the mind on this center one becomes clairvoyant. *Clairvoyant* means "to be able to see things clearly as they are." Ordinarily, one does not see things as they are and therefore becomes confused. Once the mind has become inward and one-pointed, if you steadily meditate on this tiny circle, you will find a light coming through. If there is a light in the mind's eye, follow it and try to hold it still. When it moves, observe its movements and how the mind runs away from it.

Before going to bed, sit down and focus on the space between the two eyebrows. When you focus here you can receive that which is considered to be pure knowledge. The impressions you have stored within will start coming before your mind one by one. Those impressions can disturb the beginner and distract them from their concentration.

In Upanishadic literature there are two types of impressions—*klishta* and *aklishta*—those that are helpful and those that are disturbing. Some are dormant, some you can observe and analyze and some you cannot analyze. You can allow those patterns from the unconscious that are helpful to you to come and stop those that are disturbing to you. A pleasant impression is not necessarily good, and a good impression may not always be pleasant, as darkness is not light and light is not darkness. There cannot be a compromise between the two, just as there cannot be a compromise between karma and knowledge. So you should understand not only that which is pleasant but also good, and what is pleasant and not pleasant. Sometimes a teacher's instructions may seem to be very unpleasant, so you don't want to follow them. Instead, you prefer to follow the whims of your mind and senses. That is why it is important for you to meditate. Through meditation, you can come to understand your samskaras. You all know how your past thinking, actions and emotions have made a space deep down in your unconscious mind where they remain for a long time. These are your samskaras.

When you focus your mind on the proper chakra you should decide not to identify with your thought patterns. The teachers of meditation say, "Learn to make your abode in complete darkness." It is very easy to imagine light, but it is very difficult to observe darkness and maintain that darkness for some time. A student is asked to observe complete darkness within so they can see the real light that is far away. But in no way at this point should you ever try to meditate on the crown chakra or any lower chakra. If you meditate on the crown, or sahasrara chakra, without guidance you might start to hallucinate.

For both anahata and ajna chakra, involving visualization while listening to the sound vibrations is equally helpful. But switching from one to the other is a waste of time and can be discouraging. You can receive intuitive knowledge by both ways when you practise faithfully.

GURU CHAKRA: When Patanjali says to meditate on the chakra that is below the crown, he is not talking about sahasrara, the seventh chakra. He is referring to the guru chakra, the space of the guru within. This is where the guru within, the fire of the knowledge within, dwells. It is the light of this knowledge within you that dispels the darkness. The symbol of the guru chakra is an upward triangle, a symbol of fire. As you have a navel center, manipura chakra, there is also a cavity here. The space between the eyebrows is called *bhrikuti.* But there is another that is called *trikuti. Tri* means "three." Three lines make a trikuti and this is the guru chakra. Guru chakra does not refer to the external guru. *Guru* means "knowledge" or "light."

If you meditate on the light that is within, that particular light will guide you. The external guru instructs the student to meditate on the guru chakra when they are confused and cannot find the way or when they want to solve certain problems of the inner path. When this happens, there is no need to contact the external guru. By meditating on the guru chakra, you may have a vision of those persons who are already enlightened. You may suddenly see somebody having a big beard and white robe and sitting somewhere and you don't know who it is. By chance you have come in touch with that chakra that can give you visions of perfected beings or beings in another world.

INTUITION

The finest of all knowledge is intuition, and intuitive diagnosis is the finest of all diagnostic tools, especially where other methods have failed. In order to diagnose the ailments in others, you first concentrate on the point between the two eyebrows (ajna chakra) the gateway to the city of life. Then, shift to trikuti. If your teacher teaches you to meditate on this, you can develop the ability of intuitive diagnosis. Intuitive diagnosis is a matter of concentration. I focus my one-pointed mind on the gland centers of the patient and can pinpoint the source and nature of trouble. One of the benefits of intuitive diagnosis is that you can diagnose future ailments today:

Once I went to a place called Bhiwani, which is in Haryana, one of the states of India. I visited a Sanskrit school and saw that the teacher was holding a book, *Duti Vijnanam*. *Duti* means "messenger;" *vijnanam* means "knowledge." When a messenger comes to you and tells you that something has happened to the patient, you immediately know what it is. That book gives you that knowledge. It is written in very good classical Sanskrit. I asked him if

I could borrow the book so I could read it. After the third day I returned it to him. By chance, shortly after I had arrived, the son of a patient came. "My mother is suffering on account of headache. Can you help?"

He said, "Yes. Come here." And he slapped him and said, "Go back. Your mother is all right."

I said, "I have not seen this type of doctor before."

So I followed that person until he had reached home. His mother told him the headache suddenly went off. I suspected maybe some people create such problems just for the sake of publicity. So, I took an arthritis patient to him. I advised the patient not to enter with me but to go ahead of me and I would come after ten minutes.

When she came she said, "Swamiji, I am not well. I have arthritis." All the joints were affected and they were swollen and paining. Swamiji slapped her and she became alright.

There is something beyond that also. This is a historical fact. Have you heard about Humayan and Baber in Indian history? Their story is very famous. They were kings—son and father. When the doctors declared that the son was going to die, the father was told to go around the son's bed carrying a glass of water four times. Then, he was to drink that water. The son would live and he would die. He said he was prepared to save his son because he had already lived for a long time. And so it happened. This was possible because of sankalpa shakti—full determination. All human beings have that potential.

Once you reach the state of superconsciousness, all knowledge comes forth. By concentrating on the guru chakra, you will definitely receive the knowledge that comes from the valley of intuition or pure knowledge. Eventually, you will have to even go beyond that.

PRAYER, CONTEMPLATION and MEDITATION

PRAYER
TYPES of PRAYER
SELFLESS SERVICE
LAW of KARMA
HEALING
HOW to PRAY
ARE PRAYERS ANSWERED
EXAMPLES of PRAYER
CONTEMPLATION

PRAYER, CONTEMPLATION AND MEDITATION

The great sages in the past discovered three different ways to go within: prayer, contemplation and meditation. They are all helpful, but they cannot comfort you in your daily life if your actions are scattered and misdirected. That which cannot be solved in any other way, can be solved through prayer. You contemplate on certain ideas like how to practise truth and when you concentrate your mind uninterruptedly on one point for some time, that is meditation. In prayer, you are conversing with the Lord, while meditation is more toward silence. Otherwise, there is very little difference. These are three great schools and they can all help to make you aware of the innermost center of consciousness and to attain enlightenment. The purpose of these three schools is to lead you to the fountainhead of life, love and light from which this power flows.

PRAYER

Those who cannot meditate should concentrate through prayer. But for prayer you also need to have a one-pointed mind. If you are praying to God and thinking of a glass of water, you'll get only a glass of water. If you want to create a whirlpool for yourself you can condemn and destroy yourself: *How petty I am, how bad I am, how little I am, I cannot do anything, I am of no use, nobody loves me, everybody hates me.* It is your prerogative to regress or progress. You need courage and strength from within. Don't go backward. What you have done for a few months or a few years ago is gone and finished. Don't brood on that and don't condemn yourself. Instead, repentance is good. All the great religions have the same system. For example, in Catholicism there is confession.

But you should remember that the person to whom you are confessing is not better than you; they are exactly like you with all the vices and virtues that you can imagine. So what good is your repentance? You are letting out your hidden weaknesses, bringing them to the surface so you can deal with them. If you are doing something knowingly, that is not weakness. Weakness is that which makes you a victim. *Repentance* means "you are not going to repeat it again." That is all. You did it. It is past. You are not going to do it again. You should have that strength. That is the only way to deal with samskaras so you can be free. However, if you go on repeating the same mistake many times and keep asking the Lord to forgive you, that is not the way to freedom. PRAYER AND REPENTANCE PURIFY THE WAY OF THE SOUL. If you think that you have done something that you shouldn't have done, don't repeat it and you will be free. Don't condemn yourself or tell yourself you are bad. The sense of guilt is strengthened when you go on repeating the same thing and then accept that you cannot help yourself. No matter what happens, don't accept defeat. Don't do what is not to be done and you will be free. You know from inside that you are very weak and that you have not purified yourself, yet you pose to sit in meditation or you start to pray, even though you are convinced that nobody is listening to your prayers. When you go against your conscience in this way, your inner desires, your will and your conscience slowly weaken, and you lose the finest instrument you have. Be practical and do your actions with the understanding that action is one of the finest of all prayers.

Don't worry about opposition. If you think and live like people say you should, you will not survive in this world. During Christ's time the Romans and the Jews opposed him. Similarly, many Jews opposed Moses, many

Hindus opposed Krishna and many Buddhists opposed Buddha. The more you find opposition, the more your path is clear. But while going to bed, you should remember this: *I will not repeat it again.* Suppose you repeat it? Again you will have to try. Don't give up. Sometimes failure is the pillar of success. Then, pray to the Lord: *Lord of life, who is seated beyond body, senses and mind, you know me and you are witnessing all my actions and thoughts. Give me the strength and energy so that I can fulfil the mission of life. Guide me so I do not hurt or harm anyone and am able to go through this journey without any interference.* In this way, you are coming in direct touch with the source of consciousness that gives you strength. Muscular strength is nothing, but mental strength is tremendous. Even more than that, the strength of Atman is immense!

The school of prayer is valid. Prayer gives you strength so you can easily go through this procession of life smiling, without harming, hurting or injuring anyone. You are responsible for the problems you have created for yourself, so you also have the power to get freedom from those problems. PRAYER GIVES YOU STRENGTH. Those who do not pray are weak people. Those persons who live for a cause are fearless because they have a goal in front of them. They pray to the Lord and believe in the Lord who witnesses all their actions, speech and thoughts. Prayer is a very powerful instrument, provided you know how to pray. Then you can pray for both those who are here and those who have gone. Prayer makes you aware and strengthens your awareness and determination.

TYPES of PRAYERS

There are two types of prayer: EGOCENTRIC PRAYER (*sakama prarthana, sakama upasana, sakama bhakti*) and GOD-

CENTERED PRAYER. Most of your prayers are egocentric prayers in which you are praying to your ego to satisfy your ego. You should use your ego like you use your shoes so that it wears out. Instead, you continue to feed it. You say you don't need to do meditation because you pray. However, you do not pray the way you should. Your prayers are ego-centered prayers and they cannot take you beyond. Don't pray to God for anything worldly. You are just feeding your ego and this will never improve your life. No doubt prayer has immense power, but ego-centered prayer will only make you weak. You ask God to give you this and that. That cripples you because you are begging. You become dependent when you ask for things all the time. You have formed this bad habit and you are wasting your energy for petty demands. There is no need to ask God for anything because God already knows your needs. There is a difference among needs, wants, wishes and desires. Your days are laden with wants and nights with desires, so you remain disturbed all the time. Never pray for petty things or with selfish motivation. You find yourself helpless because you do not know how to apply your means, inner strength and intelligence. When you are in trouble you become a needy person and you think that a higher power that you call God will help you. However, when everything is okay with you, you forget all about God.

Every individual has a question because life itself is a big question mark. You want that question to be answered by someone higher and greater, so you call it God. When you pray, that prayer should be God-centered prayer. I am not talking about praying to someone who is outside you and far away from you, whom you have never seen or never known. It is important to understand to which god you are praying. You should pray directly to the Lord of life who is seated deep within you in the inner chamber of your being, beyond body, breath and mind. Pray to the Self that is deep within you, who sees through your eyes, listens through your ears and motivates your whole being. Remember that your body is a shrine and the inner dweller to whom you are praying is the real deva.

God-centered prayer is higher than ego-centered prayer and will never make you weak. In God-centered prayer you do not ask for petty things. Instead you only ask for strength to face life and to understand life as it is, so that you can face all the challenges in your life. Ask the Lord to guide you and give you inner strength, and He will help you because He is within you. God-centered prayer will help you to increase your will power. He knows what is good for you, so there is no need for you to ask for anything. You just have to do your duties; the rest He knows. The sadhaka should have that confidence. You are responsible for doing your actions; don't worry for the fruits therein. Instead, pray to the Lord for strength so that you become aware of the center of consciousness from where you receive strength. *I am weak, Lord; I don't have anyone except you. Give me strength so that I can be of some service to humanity and serve others.* Go to the deeper aspects of your being, to the source from where you get energy and strength. *Prayer* means "a wish or a powerful one-pointed desire to serve others." It's that desire itself that communicates. That prayer will make you aware of the reality within you. When you are conscious of this, your whole energy will be motivated toward the desire you are praying for, and the desire will definitely be fulfilled. In addition, your awareness will be strengthened.

SELFLESS SERVICE

It's wrong to pray for health just for the sake of health. If you say, *Oh Lord, give me good health because I want to enjoy the good things of the world,* this is not a good prayer. It's better to pray for health so that you can accomplish your task of selfless service: *Give me good health so that I can help and serve others.* Those who know what selfless service is know it is the greatest of all prayers. In selfless service you don't expect anything; you just serve. That is the way for liberation. Throughout human history and civilization there have been countless individuals who have made the pilgrimage from a narrow focus on *I, me, mine* to choosing to love and serve society. As they have increasingly dedicated themselves to the benefit of humankind and the recognition of the universal consciousness in all, numerous gifts and powers have unfolded for their selflessness to help others. Great individuals like Christ, Buddha, Gandhi and others all saw themselves as instruments of the higher force of consciousness, love and power in the universe, not as petty human beings preoccupied with trivial desires and pleasures. Through selfless action you can be free all the time because you are performing your actions and giving up the fruits of your actions for others.

Many people suffer because they do not understand the importance of selfless service. *Selfless service* means "to do your actions and duties selflessly, skillfully and lovingly." You cannot convince yourself to do selfless service unless you have fully understood the law of karma. Your samskaras continue to motivate you to do selfish work and that creates more entanglement. Your individual soul creates bondage because of attachment and you are caught in the snare of those bondages. If you are not free from those bondages, you will never be happy. To get freedom from all suffering is the aim of life. This is possible when you serve others. Remember, suffering comes from relationships, so you have to deal with your relationships. You expect from the world, and the world expects from you. The world is disappointed, and you also remain disappointed.

You should understand that when you do something selflessly for someone else, you should enjoy doing that. If you think you are doing something selflessly, but your mind is actually somewhere else, then that is not really a selfless act. You are doing something half-heartedly, absentmindedly and without any true interest. Learn to enjoy things by putting your whole heart and mind into them, and then you will really enjoy them. If anything strains you, then you should realize that either your body, mind or heart does not fully agree, and that is why you are strained. What I am trying to make clear is that although you can do actions in your daily life selflessly, they may not be good for your physical and psychological health if you do not have true interest. If you do not do things wholeheartedly you will not enjoy them, no matter how much selfless action you try to do. Learn to enjoy the things you are doing for others. The highest enjoyment is what you experience when you are doing something selflessly for others yet you are at the same time enjoying it.

You can have freedom from past karmas only by transforming yourself. Selfless service is a must to get rid of the bondage of karma. The more selfless you become, the closer you come to another level of life. No one can live without doing actions, so you should live to do selfless service because that is the only way to get freedom from the bondage of karma. Humanity is suffering, because human beings are selfish. One who is selfish builds boundaries around themself that prevent them from serving others. You are not the same person you were 20 years ago because you are constantly growing. Life is a process of growth, whether you want to grow or not. You should prepare yourself for that growth so that it becomes comfortable for you. If you do not prepare, then you will remain under stress. You will find that your whole life is a process of growth, unfolding and enlightenment, but often you do not cooperate with that.

The highest human potentials are expressed by those willing to be silent and peaceful and to forgo status and power. They quietly and lovingly go about their work, teaching and helping others without expectation of reward. Thus, love and an attitude of acceptance make possible the unfolding of the higher powers and represent the dawn of a human being's growth. As they continue to evolve, still other potentials may express themselves to be put to the use of serving others. When human beings learn to fathom the deeper levels of their being, then real knowledge will dawn and they will learn to love all and exclude none. SELFLESS SERVICE IS THE WAY TO FREEDOM.

LAW OF KARMA

You might wonder what it is that motivates someone to become selfless. The law of karma is: *As you sow so shall you reap.* This is the law of action and cause and effect. You are performing actions from morning till evening and you are reaping fruits accordingly. Those fruits again motivate you to do more actions. In this way you create a whirlpool around yourself and you are not able to come out of that. You cannot escape from the law of karma. You have to do actions because you cannot live without doing them, and you have to reap the fruits, because of your actions. It seems there is no way to get freedom no matter how much you pray.

When you study the law of karma, you come to know there is only one way out and that is to renounce the fruits of your actions for the sake of others. That is real worship. One who has understood this law is free and can heal others at any distance. A selfless person who understands the law of the universe, knows that freedom comes once one becomes selfless. One who knows the law is serving the universe not for the sake of obliging others but for the sake of their own freedom. You have heard that Christ healed many times, and that all the great messengers had the capacity to heal. You have that same capacity, but you will have to come in touch with those healing potentials. It is not as difficult as you might think to control diseases. If the heart is mine, I should be able to control it. I can control any part of the body. Otherwise, I could not claim it is my body; it would be something apart from me. The power of self-healing is within every human life. By uncovering that potential not only can you heal yourself, you can heal others.

If you want to heal yourself, then you should know those principles. And if you want to heal others then you should become selfless. A completely selfless person can heal anyone. You can start through actions and speech. You can sometimes sit down and think how you can help others selflessly, especially those who are not related to you. If you are helping only those who are related to you, you might have some selfish motivation. That is not selfless service, but charity begins from home. When you learn to do charity at home then you expand your consciousness to cosmic consciousness. That is freedom. You have all the potentials and resources to attain a state of freedom from the bondages you have created for yourself. If you are lost and you think you have committed too many mistakes, then start to practise. The simplest way is to serve the people with whom you live. That is the greatest of all prayers. You can create happiness in the world by serving others according to your capacity. In selfless service, everything that is given or received is offered to the Lord. TO SERVE OTHERS IS TO SERVE THE LORD.

HEALING

With a one-pointed desire to serve selflessly, you can heal many people. No one can be selfless if they have no love for others. In today's world, the most used word is *I* and then *love*. From morning till evening you use this word *I, I, I, I.* If you identify yourself with your thought patterns, the objects of the world and your body, then that *I* will suffer. If you think *I am body,* you will definitely suffer because the body is subject to change, death and decay. On the other hand, if you understand the *I* that is the light in the lamp of life, you will have no fear. I am talking about those people who have known the mysteries of life and lead a fearless life because they understand what life is. If you really understand that *I* that is not body, senses or mind but is beyond, nothing is impossible.

The key point of healing is selflessness. If you are selfless, you really want to heal someone and you do not expect any reward, name or fame, you can do that. If someone does their work selflessly, they can have access to tremendous power. Many people think they are very powerful and can heal others. You may be successful in praying for others, but you should remember that a human being actually has no power to heal others. That power belongs only to the absolute reality. One who is aware of this fact is a humble person; one who is not aware of this suffers on account of ego problems. Many healers come in touch unconsciously with this divine power once or twice and they become egotistical and think they are channels of the Lord. They are not. ALL POWER BELONGS TO GOD. All else is vanity.

There are three levels of healing: physical, mental and spiritual. One who has spiritual power can heal others on all levels, but if he tries to make healing his profession, his mind will again start to run toward worldly grooves. A dissipated and worldly mind is not fit to heal anyone. The moment one becomes selfish, the mind changes its course and starts flowing downward to the lower grooves. Misuse of spiritual power weakens and distracts the very basis of that power, which is called *iccha shakti*. Those who are great always say that all the powers belong to the Lord and they are only instruments. Every human being has potentials for healing. The healing energy is flowing without any interruption in every human heart. By the right use of the dynamic will, these channels of healing energy can be directed to the suffering part of the body and mind. The healing energy can nourish and strengthen the sufferer. The keys to healing are selflessness, love, dynamic will and undivided devotion to the Lord within.

Not only can yogis heal themselves, they can also heal others. Mind has the capacity to cure. I have demonstrated that I could create a tumor on my body only by thinking negatively. I do it so intensely that a lump actually comes. That shows how a negative mind can immediately create problems in the body. Then, I think positively to make it disappear. Now, not everybody can do that. They can create a tumor, but they do not know how to dissolve what they have created. If mind is very strong, and it voluntarily creates a tumor, then it should also be able to dissolve it. Similarly, mind can create many varieties of cancer, strokes and heart attacks.

Pain and pleasure is a pair of opposites experienced when the senses contact objects of the world. Those whose consciousness has expanded beyond the sensory level get freedom from this pair of opposites. There are techniques for voluntarily withdrawing the mind from the senses and focusing inward to reveal the center of consciousness where you will not be affected by sensory pleasure or pain. Such a one-pointed mind also creates a dynamic will, which can then be used for healing others. All such healing powers flow through the human being from the one source of the center of consciousness within. The moment the healer becomes conscious of his individuality, that spontaneous flow of healing power will stop. Healing is a natural power in humans. The healing of others is possible through that will power which is not interrupted by the lower mind.

If you observe people, you'll conclude that most of their thinking and behavior is more negative than positive. There is nothing like negative emotion or passive emotion. Actually, these are just grooves that you create mentally. If you have a positive attitude, nothing will affect you. But if you hear something negative, you tend to think of it constantly. Don't allow negativity to influence your mind or remain under the influence of stress. Stay happy and be aware of the physician within that heals you. For a happy and healthy life, you need a comfortable environment, cheerfulness and positive thinking, and a good diet. If you eat very good food but do not know how to think positively, your biochemistry can convert your food into poisons. It is necessary for you to be cheerful to enjoy life. Never forget that cheerfulness is the biggest physician, the self-healer within you.

Will power is another means for healing. You can get freedom from all suffering and attain a state of joy and happiness. If you understand the power of positive thinking and you remain conscious of the reality within you can remain free from many diseases. I am not saying that suffering does not exist outside. There are many sources of suffering. But first of all you should learn to be free from the suffering you are creating for yourself. Then only will you have the strength to cope with the suffering you find around you and to serve and help those who are suffering. The highest of all healings is to attain freedom from all miseries.

HOW TO PRAY

Morning and evening hours are considered to be best for prayer, but you should regulate yourself. You will never have trouble if you pray rightly. I believe in prayer, but there is a difference between prayer and meditation, and there is a difference from one prayer to another.

Now, you question in which language should you pray. There is no rule that declares that prayer should be conducted in Sanskrit, Arabic, English, Latin or any other language. Prayer should be conducted in your own language, the language in which a newborn baby speaks to its mother. That is the language of love, the language of the heart. It's not important in which language you pray, but PRAYER SHOULD BE FROM THE HEART. You should pray in your own language, as silently as possible, with full determination and faith. *Oh Lord, help me attain the goal I have set. Help me to meditate.* Always pray to God to give you strength and wisdom so you can fulfill the purpose of life. *Thy will my Lord, not my will.* You are an instrument of the Lord; LET GOD PLAY THROUGH YOU.

Other people should not make prayers for you. Don't allow your mind to interfere in your prayers or you will be arguing instead of praying. Gently close your eyes and with all your feelings and thoughts ask the Lord of life to give you wisdom and strength. *O Lord, help me to be a good person. Make me thy instrument. Lord I am thine and thou art mine.* Sometimes you may pray in this manner, while other times you may open the Bible and read it. Both can help to inspire you to become spiritual and strong from within.

ARE PRAYERS ANSWERED?

Sometimes ego-centered prayers are heard and sometimes not. When your faith is intense, prayers that are rightly said are always answered. If you shoot an arrow on a target, where it hits depends on your concentration when you shot the arrow. Nothing is impossible and there is nothing that cannot be obtained through prayer, but there is one condition. If you are talking to a god that is outside you and you are ignoring the god within, your prayers will not be answered. Otherwise, all prayers are answered. No prayer ever goes in vain. If your prayer is not fulfilled it means it was half-hearted and was done under uncertainty without faith. You were not sure you were going to get whatever you were asking for. Or, maybe your prayer was something unrealistic, very selfish or at the wrong place or time. If you are churning sand to take butter out of the sand, even if you are very sincere and working very hard, you will not be successful.

Try to pray in your own language and without any doubts. Whenever you have doubts, your prayers will be only partially answered. When your mind, thoughts and emotions, are integrated and you become one-pointed, your prayers will never go in vain. In Islam it is said that once or twice a day, the individual soul should be tuned to the Lord of life. When you are meditating or praying, you are in touch with something higher. Very few people know how to take advantage of that moment.

EXAMPLES OF PRAYERS

GAYATRI MANTRA is an ancient Sanskrit mantra with multiple spiritual benefits: healing on all levels, purification, protection and Self-realization.

Om bhur bhuva swaha
Tat savitur varenyam
Bhargo devasya dhimahi
Dhiyo yo nah prachodayat.

"Divine mother, please let your pure, spiritual
and divine energy spread through all the realms
present around me and light up all the beings
present over here. Please remove any darkness
from my nature and fill me with knowledge."

All Upanishadic prayers lead you to awareness. Actually, they are not prayers; they are verses for contemplation, though they are called prayers. This is the prayer of self-awareness. It makes you aware that you can dive deep into the innermost center where peace, happiness and wisdom dwell.

Asato ma Sadgamaya,
tamaso ma jyotir gamaya,
mrtyor ma amritam gamaya.

Lead me from the unreal to the real.
Lead me from darkness to light.
Lead me from mortality to immortality.

Three desires are expressed in this prayer:

LEAD ME FROM THE UNREAL TO THE REAL.

Here, the unreal means this apparent reality
that seems to be real but is not absolutely real.
Lead me from this to the ultimate truth.

LEAD ME FROM DARKNESS TO LIGHT.

Dispel all the ignorance that has been created
by my karma, mind, action and speech. Here,
darkness means ignorance. You suffer on account of
ignorance. Buddha said avidya is the mother of all
problems. You should be free from this ignorance
you have created by your actions, thinking and
understanding.

LEAD ME FROM MORTALITY TO IMMORTALITY, MY LORD.

So far you are aware of the mortal aspect of life.
Someone is born, they grow, become a young person,
go to old age and then die. When a human being
dies, then you do not know what happens. There is
another aspect of life that is called immortality.

Oh Lord, from this worldly awareness,
guide me to the highest spiritual awareness.

The following is another example of a prayer that can help you to improve yourself and deepen your awareness:

Oh Lord of life, you are within me. Help my mind to understand the way to conduct my duties so I can become successful in the world, yet remain non-attached. If I become attached to the things of the world, I will forget the reality of life. Make me aware of this and help me to strengthen my mind, oh Lord.

When you pray in this way you prepare your mind and all the levels of your being for the inner experience of meditation.

CONTEMPLATION

From here you will find two different schools: the school of contemplation and the school of meditation. The goal of both is to attain the absolute truth. There are eight steps on both the paths of contemplation and meditation. The first goal is freedom from all fear, the second is freedom from pain, the third is freedom from all misery, the fourth is to be aware of your conscience, the fifth is to be aware of the light, the sixth is to tread the path of light within, the seventh is contentment and the eighth goal is attainment.

In the school of contemplation there is a system. You have to listen to your teacher who has been taught by the tradition and you have to study the sayings and finest parts of the scriptures. Once you have done that, you can start to contemplate on truth: *There is only one Self-existent truth here, there and everywhere that is omnipresent, omniscient and omnipotent.* However, you cannot be liberated by knowing alone. You also have to practise truth with mind action and speech. If you commit a blunder or mistake in practising truth, by the quest of truth you will be corrected and brought back to the path.

In your daily life, if you use the process of contemplation during the whole day, your work will not suffer. On the other hand, meditation needs an object that is subtle and fine. Without an object, you cannot meditate. You should not change the object of focus of meditation again and again. If you choose a particular object you should not after some time change it to another. That would be like trying to reach a destination and then changing the route every day. You would never reach there! So, the object of meditation must be constant.

Human beings are suffering because there are millions of objects in their mind. This is why the mind is distracted and runs in the many grooves of those objects. For example, perhaps you love someone. If you start to love someone else also, there will be a division in your thinking and behavior. Something similar will happen if you have many objects of meditation. This is why there should be only one object of meditation. The sages had an object of meditation and besides that they would contemplate the whole day. You also can easily contemplate the whole day. Select one issue every day, for example, I will not lie. In this way you can observe your strength. Ask yourself, *Let me see who is stronger. Am I strong, or are the people around me stronger? Are they forcing me to lead my life the way they want? Am I strong enough to lead my life the way I want, even though I'm living in the world?*

It's very easy not to lie if there is no one to whom you must speak truth. You can easily go to live in a monastery and remain in silence.

Prayer is complementary to meditation, it does not oppose meditation. First you should pray, then meditate and in the end comes contemplation.

DHYANA

SUTRA 2: *Tatra pratyaikatanata dhyanam.*
UNINTERRUPTED FLOW OF THE MIND TOWARD
ITS OBJECT IS MEDITATION.

MEDITATION DEFINED
IS MEDITATION SUITABLE for YOU
EXPECTATIONS
BENEFITS
MEDITATION and RELIGION
MEDITATION as THERAPY
PSYCHOSOMATIC DISEASE
MEDITATION in ACTION

MEDITATION DEFINED

The English translation of the Sanskrit word *dhyana* is "meditation," but this does not convey the exact meaning. Actually, the word *meditation* has not been defined properly in any of the English dictionaries. According to the dictionaries, the word *meditation* means "contemplation" and *contemplation* means "meditation." Even in the Bible the word meditation has not been thoroughly explained. *Meditation* actually means "to attend to something with full devotion and commitment." Or as Patanjali describes it in the second aphorism of *Vibhuti Pada*, UNINTERRUPTED FLOW OF THE MIND TOWARD ITS OBJECT IS MEDITATION.

Concentration is not meditation; it is only a beginning stage of meditation. While concentration can lead to strain, meditation leads to relaxation. In concentration, the mind flies here and there and then comes back; dhyana is intense, one-pointed awareness. When attention flows in one direction without interruption, then it becomes meditation. *Dharana* means "to make the mind one-pointed;" *dhyana* means "to expand that one-pointed mind to universality." So dharana is narrowing down; dhyana is expansion. That expansion should lead you to the eternal, to samadhi.

When Patanjali is talking about prayer and meditation, he is not talking about something that is outside you. He is talking about the finest part of you that is within you. You know your body, senses and mind, but you have not known the best part of yourself. You are not yet aware that there are many internal states of mind and levels of consciousness and many planes of experience. Meditation is a system that leads you beyond your body, senses, breath, conscious mind, unconscious mind and then to the center of consciousness that is the source of light and life within you. Meditation is an inward method that opens new dimensions for you and helps you to experience the highest levels of consciousness. To become aware of the subtler levels of your life and the finest level of your being, you will have to learn the method of meditation. THE SECRET OF LIFE IS REVEALED IN MEDITATION IN SILENCE.

All great traditions have come from one source and that is truth. To know truth, you have to know your finest Self. MEDITATION INTRODUCES YOU TO YOUR FINEST SELF and makes you aware of the source of love, light and life that is within. Meditation is a method of going inward, from the grossest to the subtlest aspects of your being. Meditation gives you direct experience.

You all try to be philosophers without having a system to follow. Before you try to create a philosophy you should find a way to study and understand the individual that you are, because no one else can do that for you. Meditation is a technique supported by a philosophy of life that is independent of all other philosophies. If you really want to know yourself and understand your internal states, then you should systematically tread the path. The technique of meditation can help you to know yourself and build the philosophy you need. Later, you can study the different philosophies of the East and the West to help you to know how to relate with the universe and with other individuals. Those philosophies will be helpful to understand the mysteries of life here and hereafter, and how this universe has come into existence. But first, you must know yourself. Meditation means to turn the mind inward to fathom the deeper levels of your being, instead of being involved in day to day problems. Meditation is an inward method that helps you to systematically go from one level to another and to know the latent part of your life so you can face it. If you keep running away from yourself and trying to escape from the realities of life, you are only denying yourself. The more you know yourself, the closer you will be to the Lord of life. Without knowing yourself you cannot know the Self of all. Still today at the gate of the Delphi it is written KNOW THYSELF. It has not been written to know God. First, you should understand what you are before trying to understand what God is. There is no need to worry for God because you are already God! Now, you have to learn to be human. Once you know yourself, you can know the Self of all. And for knowing yourself, nothing external can help you. But there is a way, and that is meditation, a journey without movement. In all journeys you keep moving, but in this journey you don't move and yet you go forward.

The best thing I have learned in my life is meditation. If you meditate, you will never be lonely. No one can ever make you happy if you are not happy yourself; nobody can give you company if you are not company to yourself. If you know yourself you will be able to better relate with your family and friends. All relationships can be transformed into means. This way you will better understand yourself and will be able to communicate more effectively with others. By interacting with others you learn how to live in the external world, but your inner world remains unknown to you. You are a stranger to yourself and when you meet someone for the first time it is as if you are introducing a stranger to a stranger. This is why there is great confusion in the world and so many problems in communication and relationships. The more you know yourself the more comfortable you will be in the world. You are trying to relate and communicate with others without understanding why you think and behave the way you do. You have to understand yourself first and then you will have no problem in communicating with others.

It is easy to adjust to the external world, but it is not so easy to understand the Self within, because your thoughts, emotions, desires and appetites can lead you in many different directions. When your mind is distracted, it is even more powerful and can be very destructive. In meditation, mind becomes one-pointed and inward. Only a pure mind can attain one-pointedness. Such a mind has immense capacity. For attaining any object in the world you need a one-pointed mind, and then everything will be at your disposal. You worry that your mind is running here and there and you exhaust yourself trying to control the mind. Meditation is a way to train your mind to follow a particular path and to be with you wherever you are. Mind already has a way of running, so it is best to let it run free, but according to your wishes. Sit down and let your mind go, and it will eventually come back. If you study mind you will come to know it is a characteristic of mind to have many thoughts, like the waves in the ocean. A thought comes, followed by another thought and then another. Between every two thoughts there is a space. If you could expand the space that is between two thoughts, that would be meditation. If there were only one thought, what would happen to that space?

Meditation is a method of self-inquiry, self-understanding and self-analysis that ultimately leads to self-control and self-enlightenment. Thus, meditation is a technique that helps one to experience the higher levels of consciousness. You cannot understand the center of consciousness, the source of infinite love, through the mind, because the center of consciousness is beyond mind. Though mind is a great tool, it is not capable of knowing anything beyond the level of mind. No matter how efficient your telescope is, if you turn that telescope toward yourself, it won't help you. Likewise, the glasses that you use to read help you to study, but if you turn those glasses toward you, they will not show you your internal states. You have to go beyond mind. You do not need any external instrument to know truth, because it is self-existent.

Meditation is a subjective practice, a state wherein the mind closely examines the object upon which it is concentrating. This is the power to discriminate, the power of differentiation and the first stage of liberation from action. It can only be attained through intense mental training, consisting of consciously and involuntarily identifying one's self with something or with a state of being. One must be aware of the object of meditation and the thought that is operative at the time, as well as the various stages of consciousness through which it passes. By stilling the body, making the breath serene, calming the conscious mind and next the unconscious mind, you will be there at the center of consciousness.

It is said, *Dhyanam nirvishayam manah.* Meditation is a method that can help your mind get freedom from all disturbances and obstacles. Your so-called god is left behind and you move on. This means if you follow the system of meditation faithfully, you will finally experience the formless.

Meditation can make you very creative. To be creative means to use your knowledge in time as it is needed. It is a positive method that can be used for leading a creative life and becoming successful in the world while maintaining tranquillity within. With the aid of meditation the aspirant experiences higher levels of life and is able to realize all creative potentials in the rush and roar of modern civilization. The simple and natural process of directing the mind within enables one to lead thoughts, emotions and desires to the center of reality. It is a unique method that helps you to establish yourself in your essential nature beyond visions, sounds and so-called psychic experiences. Meditation is not a passive method. It is not something negative nor is it a goofy method that makes you hallucinate. The purpose of meditation is to give you the experience of higher levels of consciousness. MEDITATION IS A VERY POWERFUL THING.

IS MEDITATION SUITABLE FOR YOU?

I have never told you that meditation means to cripple your life by withdrawing from the world. You don't have to stop doing your duties or leave your home or renounce your family. I am not saying you should not enjoy the world or you should renounce the world. That path is meant only for a fortunate few. You don't have to become a swami to qualify to practise meditation. You just have to be aware in all situations and depend on your inner strength, not on external strength. Learn to appreciate and admire yourself and become aware of the potentials within. Then, you can express those positive potentials to help you understand the external world.

You may sit and pose for meditation but if you neglect your duties your mind will bring all those things before you. Then, instead of meditating you will be thinking about all the things you have to do. Don't ignore your duties in the external world or become inert and useless, because then you will become a burden to yourself and others. Let your family know that you meditate at a certain time. Arrange your situation in a way so there are no obstacles from your family life, your social life and your economical life, and then you will be free to meditate.

Vivekananda wrote a book in which he talks about Bhavahari Baba, who lived near Ghazipur. I rarely say his name, but the first thing I do when I sit to meditate is to mentally bow to him. He was a man of the world, not a swami. I am telling you this so you understand it is not necessary for you to become a swami to learn meditation. One who meditates is in peace when they are in silence, and also when they are doing their duties. That peace they can emanate to others.

Meditation should become a part of your daily life. For a long time without any break, you should routinely practise every day at the same time. As you eat, sleep and do your other duties, you should do meditation. It is just as important for you to meditate as it is for you to breathe. You haven't trained yourself in meditation because you thought it was something foreign or strange. Actually, meditation is a necessity of human life, just as food nourishes the body and many external pleasures act as simple consolations. If you do not meditate you will be missing something and it will be difficult for you to remain balanced. Without meditation, you cannot bring forward the inner wealth from the infinite library within to the external world so you can help others.

If you don't have the right attitude when you sit for meditation, you will feel disturbed. If you are disturbed, it means you are trying to meditate without understanding what meditation is, or you are not convinced that you should be doing meditation. You do not want to sit down quietly because you are not certain that when you do so you will have peace. If you do not convince yourself, sitting down without understanding why you are sitting will make you like a train that does not move. Still, sitting for some time is not bad. It doesn't accomplish much, but it's better than nothing. Before you begin to meditate you should understand what meditation means to you, why you want to meditate and what expectations you have of meditation.

EXPECTATIONS

Many of you complain that you meditate for two hours every day yet you have not progressed. How is it possible that you are frequently doing something and there is no reaction? It's a scientific law that for any action you perform there is a reaction. The law of karma stated simply is: AS YOU SOW, SO SHALL YOU REAP. If you are meditating why are you not getting the fruits of your actions? There must be something wrong in your technique. If your meditational technique is not complete, let me assure you, you cannot go far with it. I'm not going to believe you no matter how much you try to convince me that meditation doesn't help you. You claim you have been remembering your mantra for ages, but nothing has happened. You say you are not getting any results so there is no point in doing meditation. From the very beginning you have been committing a mistake in thinking you have been doing meditation. Sitting quietly is sitting quietly; attending the breath is attending the breath. Why do you call it meditation? You say you have been meditating for many years, but I say you have not been meditating. Many of you use meditation to escape from something unpleasant and then you complain you are not getting any results. It could also be that you do not have enough knowledge about the technique of meditation or the process of meditation. Or perhaps you are committing some mistake. If you constantly create problems for yourself in the external world, and then in the evening you sit down to meditate, that is only escape. You say you meditate but I don't think you understand what the purpose of meditation is. This is why you become discouraged after a few days and decide it's not important for you. If you are not successful it is because when you sit for meditation you are thinking and not doing meditation. If you were practising a systematic method of meditation you would not be so much in touch with the negative part of your life. First, try to understand what the reality is and face the reality instead of trying to escape from it. When you sit to meditate you will find that images and thoughts of whatever is happening to you in the external world will dominate your meditation. You are posing to meditate, but that is not meditation, because you have not done the preliminaries. Mind needs freedom, joy, peace and confidence for meditation. If you are sincerely meditating, you will certainly be benefited even though you may not be seeing it. However, if you do something half-heartedly you cannot expect good results. You should learn to wait patiently for the seeds to produce the fruits.

You see the result of actions that you perform in the world in your life, but meditation is an internal method. You are not aware that the impressions of the mantra are being stored in the unconscious. As you do actions in the external world and get some fruits from those actions, meditation gives fruits internally. Therefore, you should see the reaction internally, not externally. The more you go within yourself to the deeper levels of your being, the more you will come in touch with the reality. When mind again becomes introverted and you start thinking of the same things, that is not meditation. If you become aware of the higher reality, it will definitely help you. THE REALITY WILL LEAD YOU TO THE TRUTH.

Another problem is related to your expectations. You expect to have experiences and you complain you are not seeing anything during meditation. Students often have expectations and they want to visualize or experience strange things or have visions. You shouldn't expect to see something during meditation or have predetermined ideas about what is supposed to happen during meditation. They mistakenly think that a muscle spasm or a warm bottom signifies the awakening of the kundalini. Meditation is not something to be approached anxiously or emotionally, nor is its objective to experience unusual visions or sounds. Such predetermined imaginations may bring forth the anticipated visions, but they are in fact hallucinations and obstructions that interfere with your spiritual growth. You should thank God if you don't see anything. You already see many things outside so why should you see things when you are doing meditation? Seeing is seeing, it is not meditation. Your mind will not hallucinate and thought patterns will not disturb your meditation if you gradually lead your mind step by step. You fantasize about your goal and so you are torturing yourself. When mind is focused in the external world, you are not aware of the sound of your heartbeat, but when mind becomes quiet and more inwardly concentrated, suddenly you can hear the sound of the heartbeat and the music that is constantly going on in the brain. As the mind becomes quieter, you will be able to hear the subtle music that accompanies the movement of the breath. Eventually, when you are in a deep state of meditation you can go beyond that and become aware of the celestial sounds within.

Mind can imagine, but imagination is not meditation. If you are imagining an image and you are brooding on an image you have seen in the past, that is not meditation. Your imagination is based on impressions or images within. Patanjali says your imagination is full of fantasies and leads you to sloth and sleep. It brings back all the impressions that have been disturbing you. When I see a photograph, immediately I might think of another photograph but I will never think of the image of a donkey. There has to be some relation between the two images. Even in your haphazard thinking, there is a relationship.

Don't set up an unrealistic goal for yourself or expect to be enlightened in three months' time. First, you should see the condition of your mind. If it is a mess, it might take more time. You fix up a date and time for yourself because Swami Rama said you could be enlightened in six months' time. Then, after six months, you become upset because you are not enlightened. If you want to know and understand yourself on all levels, you have to meditate. If from the very beginning you systematically lead this path, it will not be difficult. It becomes easy for one to lead a path if that path has milestones, so that you know how far you have come and how far you have to go. You have to understand this is an entirely new venture for the mind, so you have to give some time to your mind to adapt. Mind runs very easily with the help of the senses to the external world. Now, you want to lead your mind toward the unknown without any images, forms or names.

Don't have any false expectations from meditation, because it will not give you what you expect. Don't fantasize, because that is not meditation. If you fantasize while you are sitting to meditate, you are wasting your time and energy. If there is no disturbance, then you are in meditation. The signs and symptoms of meditation are calmness, happiness and bliss. THERE IS NO MYSTERY IN IT. LET THAT WHICH IS WITHIN COME TO YOU; LET IT BE REVEALED TO YOU.

You have vast potentials within you, exactly like a hidden mine. Sometimes you are successful, sometimes you are not. But if you are a good miner you are not disappointed because you know your work. It is not necessary that wherever you dig a mine you will find gold, nor pearls wherever you dive. First, you find out where the pearls are located and then you dive. Success and failure have no meaning as far as the path and inner enlightenment are concerned. Those who are bewildered and disappointed in the study of the Self claim there is nothing in meditation. There is definitely something and it is within you. Don't accept defeat from yourself. No matter how much your neighbors, family members and friends want to help you, if you have accepted defeat from within, you have lost everything in life. Courage is the first quality that you need. Always have courage.

BENEFITS OF MEDITATION

Now, I will explain to you a few important benefits of practising meditation. When you practise systematically, the benefits of meditation are immense. The technique of meditation has proven beneficial to people in all walks of life. For example, a student who cannot concentrate and whose attention is easily dissipated will find meditation helpful. For executive stress and for those who suffer on account of insomnia, hypertension, ulcers and other kinds of psychosomatic diseases, meditation serves to relieve the stress. For the wife and mother who must cope with an inexhaustible series of roles and demands, meditation becomes an energizing companion to help restore inner peace, calmness and harmony.

Meditation will give you relaxation of the physical body, the nervous system and the mind and can help you to keep your nervous system strong. Many diseases are diseases of the nervous system. For example, psoriasis is considered to be a disease of the skin, but actually, it is a disease of the nervous system that is reflected on the skin. If you learn to calm your nervous system, it can be cured.

Nowadays, there is a serious weakness among teachers and gurus. They put a brand on meditation using their name and disturb the whole system. Meditation is meditation. It should lead you beyond body, senses, breath, conscious mind, unconscious mind and then to the center of consciousness, the source of light and life within you. If you follow the system, you will never go wrong. But if you jump from one thing to another, I am not responsible. You have to train yourself. When you meditate, all the impressions of your meditation will definitely affect you mentally. Meditation will help you to have inner strength so you can be self-reliant. Others can only inspire and guide you, but self-training depends on your own efforts. Don't be disappointed with yourself or give up. You have all the potentials, energy and intelligence to help you to improve. Be patient with yourself. A time will come when you will live in the world doing things perfectly, yet you will not be involved. You have to fathom the boundaries of the ordinary mind by persistence.

Meditation can lead you to the reality within. Because of that reality you have intelligence, you can think and understand; you can see, walk and do things. Once you have realized the reality within, you can never be harsh to anyone or hurt anyone. When you understand there is only one proprietor that is supplying energy to everyone, you will not be able to hurt or injure anyone. Violence and anger take away your reasoning power. Power is gentle; power is love. Don't waste your power in violence and negative thinking. Nonviolence is the expression of true love. You will understand what love and duty mean. Your duties will no longer feel like a burden to you, so duty will not bind you. Then, duty will become a sort of prayer for you. Just experiment and see what happens.

Self-transformation is possible through meditation, because all your activities are governed by your thoughts. You can completely transform the way you are thinking and behaving today. The relationship of wife changes into mother, and mother's relationship changes into divinity. The following are two examples of this transformation:

There was one sage in Bengal whose name was Goranganath Prabhu. He was a great man who kept chanting whenever he was awake and even while he was in deep sleep. He was so handsome that beautiful women used to follow him wherever he went.

So one day, a woman thought she would quietly hide herself under his bed at night so she might have a chance to sleep with him.

She knew that whenever he was in his room, his disciple would close the door. So there she laid herself under the cot. She could hear him constantly chanting *Hari Krishna Govinda* from his bed, and she became entranced. So, instead of trying to seduce Goranganath Prabhu, she remained in a heightened state the whole night. In the morning, she came out from beneath the cot. When that sage saw the woman he was quite surprised and asked her, "Who are you?"

She replied, "I am your mother."

She had been completely transformed.

Saradamata was the wife of Ramakrishna Paramahansa, Vivekananda's guru. Ramakrishna Paramahansa was deeply intoxicated in bhava samadhi, ecstasy. They did not have a usual husband-wife relationship. You must be thinking that he had spoiled that woman's life and wondering why they got married. However, you should be aware there was another aspect.

When he was 35 years of age his wife was only three years of age. He talked to his guru, and his guru and he both agreed. He said, "My wife was born in such and such place." So his father went to the girl's house and her father also knew. However, by the time she had grown up, he had become too old, so they never had any sort of physical relationship. They were a naturally divine couple. It means one can live in the world as householders without having a physical relationship. This is a singular example.

There was a fixed time for her to bring something for her husband, so she brought water. He was a devotee of the Mother Divine, so when he saw a woman coming he would say, "Oh, Mother, come!"

She replied, "Ai, beta." (Oh, son, I have come).
So they treated each other like mother and son
throughout their life together.

MEDITATION AND RELIGION

There is no need to put a brand on meditation—this is Christian meditation, that is Hindu meditation and that is Buddhist. Meditation is meditation. Don't think that meditation is something only for Asians or that meditation is not part of Christianity. Christians have forgotten the great wisdom of the fathers of the desert who were able to survive only with the help of the practice of meditation. Although the desert fathers were great meditators, somehow that noble tradition has been lost in Christianity. Today, many Christians even say meditation is evil and is bad for you. Whereas the Bible says the kingdom of God is within, the yogi practises to attain samadhi and Vedanta says you have to attain the absolute truth within, they all are saying one and the same thing. The different religions use different terms to describe this state, but the meaning is the same. When you study life with clarity of mind you will find that deep within you there is a center that is called the kingdom of God. The ultimate reality referred to as God by religionists, and the absolute truth according to philosophers are one and the same. He who is described as Christ in the Bible is called Krishna in the Bhagavad Gita, or Buddha. I have never been confused about this. Those great persons who have had profound influences on humanity for centuries are universal. They do not belong to anyone or to any particular religion; they belong to the universe. You will know them and love them when you become universal. You project a limited personality on them because your mind is limited.

There are two different paths. The way of the religionist is to seek the help of the grace of God for enlightenment and happiness. All the religions of the world want to have the grace of God to be happy in life. But the path of the sages is entirely different than this. Their search does not start from the idea of finding God. Their way is the recognition that we all have pain, misery and fears. They accept that pain in life exists on three dimensions: pain coming from others, from within and from outside. To them, the highest state is the state that is free from pain and misery.

First of all, you should convince yourself that meditation is not against your religion or your culture. Then only can you do meditation. Meditation is an inward method found in all the great religions of the world. If you want to meditate it does not mean you have to change your religion or your culture. To understand truth you don't have to follow any particular religion. There is meditation in Christianity and in Judaism. Meditation is an inward method. When Christ became perfect he did not become Buddhist. Likewise, when Buddha became perfect he did not become Christian. Everyone is aiming for the same height of perfection.

The philosophy I follow has been condensed from the Upanishads, Buddhism, Christianity, Judaism and Sufism. It took me a long time to assimilate all of these. It you study the Upanishads you will come to know they do not talk about God. It's the same in Buddhism, because there's no difference between Buddhist philosophy and the Upanishads. Likewise, there is no difference in the monastic way of living in Christianity, Hinduism or Buddhism. This is because the fundamentals of truth are one and the same in all religions. It is the human mind that has created the differences. It is true that every human being should build their own philosophy, and that philosophy should come through experience. You can gain that experience only when you practise. With this system you can go to the higher realms within. You should be confident of yourself and fully aware that this method of meditation will not disturb your religion or cultural concepts, but it will help you to better understand religion. Let your body become still, comfortable and steady; let your mind become still and ALLOW THE GODLY PART TO BE REVEALED TO YOU.

MEDITATION AS THERAPY

Meditation is the best of all therapies, but some people are not prepared for it. That preparation starts with having good food habits, adequate exercise and an understanding of your relationships with others. You can discard your obstinacy, become gentle with others and at the same time do your duties in life. After you meditate, you cannot then come out and give a bit of your mind to your partner. In this way, meditation is very good for wife and husband's relationship and also for father and children's relationship. There is a great gap between growing children and parents these days. The mistake lies with the parents and not the children. The parents want to control their children, but the children want to be free to grow.

Meditation is therapeutic. Many diseases can be cured, heart problems can be solved and conflicts can be resolved with the help of meditation. If you learn to be still, you can prevent many diseases. If you sit down quietly, your muscles, both voluntary and involuntary, take rest during that time. When you breathe in a serene way, the intake of oxygen and release of carbon dioxide are regulated. Meditation calms the mind, relieves muscular, nervous and mental tension, regulates metabolism and gradually brings it into balance and harmony.

Meditation helps one to have a balanced mind, which is the very basis of success in the life. Another point is that meditation provides you with an opportunity to restore the harmony between body and mind. You no longer need to feel the mental and physical fatigue that is a result of disorganized and dissipated energy. Through meditation you can regain both energy and proper perspective.

In modern times you need meditation to help you release tension and stress. You often become tense and feel drained from the day's problems. Even so-called success in the world accumulates tension, so that life seems to be a series of conflicting thoughts and stressful events. When you cannot find a solution to your problems, first you go to the bathroom. When you are not successful at solving your problems in the bathroom, then you go to sleep and you dream. Even while dreaming you cannot handle your problems so you start to snore and sleep more deeply. It is not therapeutic to try to forget your problems or to suppress or avoid them. Sooner or later you will have to deal with them. When you go to the higher states you will find greater problems, so don't think your problems will be over when you meditate. Instead, you will become more aware of your problems and how to remove them. It is better to deal with your problems consciously and fearlessly. Always try to understand why you are afraid and don't allow your will power to be weakened.

Determine that you will not have fear. You can never be fearless if you are not here and now. A time will come when the conscious mind becomes afraid of crossing that boundary. This is a good sign that you are meditating. When there is some pleasantness it means you are attaining something, so don't be afraid. You should have no fear, because you are a wave of bliss in the vast ocean of the universe and you are always protected.

Is meditation a complete therapy or do you need a therapist on whom you can lean for many years and still not understand yourself? No therapist in the world can claim to be perfect, and if the therapist is not perfect, then there is no chance that they can make you perfect. At some point you will realize you have to be independent and not lean on external crutches; YOU HAVE TO BE YOUR OWN THERAPIST. Meditation is a method of self-training. Self-transformation is possible when you become serious and are ready for therapy, and then your therapist can help you. In self-therapy you are your own therapist, but you have to be honest with yourself and practise within your capacity. If you want to work with yourself to know and understand yourself on all levels, then meditation is the only way to do that. If you know how to deal with your conscious mind and don't allow your unconscious mind to disturb the conscious mind, meditation is therapeutic.

The school of meditation says that you have to go beyond mind, to a state of tranquillity and equilibrium. Once you attain that contentment, you can easily adjust to the external world and fulfill the purpose of life. If you expect to find something other than contentment, you will be lost on the path of meditation. But if you want to be a good human being and attain perfection, then meditation is a form of self-therapy that can help you to know yourself on all dimensions and levels.

PSYCHOSOMATIC DISEASE

For years I have tried to understand the entire human mechanism, and why people suffer from disease. I have come to the conclusion that most diseases are sown in childhood. Children become ill because they have not learned the means of acquiring peace of mind. In today's schools children study the brain, but they do not learn that the mind is different from the brain. They have yet to know that greater part of mind that is beneath consciousness. Until they learn to utilize that vast portion of their mind they will remain deprived. Although the wealth is there they do not know in which corner it is buried.

Except for the few diseases that are considered to be infectious or viral diseases, most diseases are self-created and come from your mind and your emotional body, not from your soul. External tension can create many impressions in your unconscious mind that can cause disease. They are called psychosomatic diseases. Psychosomatic diseases are more powerful than physical diseases. Your emotional body is like a fish in the ocean of life that is constantly in turmoil because it is being tossed all the time. Neither emotions nor psychosomatic diseases are independently born in the unconscious. Rather they come from the impressions stored in your unconscious from your relationships in the external world. When there are psychosomatic diseases, this means there is something wrong somewhere in your relationships. And when you study your emotions you will come to know that not a single emotion is independent. Any emotion that is creating problems for you is related to someone else. If you have a healthy mind, it will protect you from many illnesses. Those who have a healthy mind get well soon, whereas others may take a long time.

Psychosomatic diseases can be healed very easily if you understand how the mind functions. The source of many diseases is conflict within and without. If you have many conflicts within, those conflicts are constantly blasting your body and your nervous system, and you suffer. Once you have a better understanding of your internal states, you will come to know that not only are you creating problems for yourself you also have inherent healing agents that are working to heal you. Many of you get sick today because of your irregular habits and then you want to be healed. You put the blame on God because you think He makes you suffer. You pray to God to make you free of misery. God neither punishes nor rewards; He simply witnesses. If you really want to know who has created misery for you, you'll find out that you have created it yourself. It is your karma that rewards or punishes you. You are suffering not because nature or God wants you to suffer. First of all, there is no reason you should be ill. If you lead a regulated life, you can prevent illness. You do not need to be healed if you are not sick. When you see physical diseases are simple, you go deeper and find that mental diseases are more serious. No matter how much you try, still they persist. You may eliminate one disease, but then another disease comes, because you do not know how to think properly. You are suffering because of your own follies.

It is not difficult at all to be healthy; you just have to decide you want to be healthy. When your unconscious is in control, your actions become automatic and you move because your unconscious makes you move. Unless you know something about your unconscious mind and have found a way to train it, you cannot be successful. In order to come to know your unconscious habits you will have to first study your conscious habits. Those who are stubborn may not want to change their habits. Even after they have become conscious of their habits they say it's difficult or impossible to change habits at an advanced age.

Even though your mind is going through a thinking process, it seems you are not progressing. This may be due to your habits that play a great role in your life. Because you do not know how to create a joyous mind, your mind roams and habitually flows to the deep grooves of the habits you have been creating your whole life. Habits are formed when you keep doing things unconsciously over and over. Habits create deep grooves and mind flows to those grooves spontaneously and unconsciously. Many habits are not helpful and could be damaging because they don't allow you to grow. Every day your mind travels through the same grooves. In addition, those feelings and thoughts and habit patterns that are reflected through your body are there. Habit patterns are strong motivations in your life, and it is not easy to break them. To have a habit means you know you should not do something, yet you are unable to stop. Many times you know that doing something is not good yet you do it, because your mind leads you to the grooves of your habits. These are old habits and you do not know how to change them. For example, you take too much alcohol even though you know it's not good for you, because it is very difficult to break that habit.

Disease can come from three main sources: hurry, curry and worry. There is a vast difference among worrying, thinking and meditating. If you have conflict you cannot make a decision. And if the mind is not under control and is not properly guided and directed, you will do everything in a disorganized and hurried manner. In addition, if you eat too much of the wrong things too fast, you will become ill. Likewise, it is not healthy to worry because worries reflect in your body as diseases. Worry cripples all aspects of your internal states — manas, chitta, buddhi and ahankara. You worry about the future and what is going to happen to you. You worry about what will happen to your partner and your children if you die. It is a waste of time and energy to worry about the future. Your personality is made up of your habits. Habit means to repeat something again and again. So first you do it consciously, but then that conscious habit becomes unconscious and you have no control over it. Only the impressions of those worries that you are interested in remain in a latent state in the bed of memories. If you could know your past lives, you would find your whole past was full of worries, but you are still alive and smiling. Many people develop the tendency to be unhealthy, sad and miserable until they create that kind of personality for themselves. There are people that love to worry and cannot live without worrying so they form a habit. That habit can be broken only by creating new grooves. Then, the mind can leave the old grooves and travel in the new grooves. The student should get up in the morning and do some exercise and breathing practices. If they have a schedule they will have no time to worry. And if unconsciously they still worry, there is a method that can slowly break those unconscious habits. Train yourself not to be affected by worries. Worrying definitely leads to suffering and consumes your energy.

Actually, there is very little difference between meditation and worry. Both control your mind, guide and direct you. The difference is worry is unconscious and negative, while meditation is positive and requires conscious effort. In addition, those who do not understand the whole technique of meditation may start to think negatively. You cannot enjoy anything if you continue to worry and it becomes a disastrous habit. It is better to know with certainty what meditation is and how meditation can help you. You think you have come to this world to stay forever and the whole world is yours. And so, you are afraid of losing it and you worry. You cannot ignore the fact that you have come for some time only, and there is very little time at your disposal, so you should enjoy. Mind control cannot prevent you from worrying but it can help you to channel and modify your worries. Everyone has worries, but they don't have to affect you.

If you pay more attention to what you are doing, you will not be under the control of your unconscious habits. There is one easy way to change habit patterns and transform the personality. When you are doing something you know isn't helpful you should do something different. Repeated actions will create new grooves in your mind to form new and more helpful habits. You have to train your mind to flow to the new grooves, from negative to positive and from passive to active. If you can work with your habits, you can enjoy total physical, mental and spiritual health.

MEDITATION IN ACTION

There are two types of meditation; meditation in silence in a quiet, remote place like a dark cave, and meditation right in the midst of your daily actions. Both meditation in silence and meditation in action are important. Of these, the secluded type of meditation may be right for the individual yogi, but it does not do much good for society. You must aim therefore at a meditation that you can practise while you are engaged in your daily chores.

The practice of sitting in meditation is preparation for meditation in action in which you express your love through your speech and actions in external life. By sitting in meditation, you become aware of the Lord's presence within you. In meditation in action you practise in your daily life by remaining aware of the reality all the time, wherever you go and whatever you do. You continue to do your duties, yet you understand the purpose of your life. You are not lost and you do not identify with the work that you do. You meet your friends, you look after your partner and your children, you go to your job and you come home, yet you are always aware of the reality. Wherever you go, you should always remain aware that the Lord is witnessing your actions.

The finest part of meditation is to apply it in daily action. You can meditate while you are doing your daily actions and your work. Meditation means to attend to whatever you are doing and not to bother with what is happening elsewhere. If you do meditation in action and always remain aware of the center of consciousness within, you will be in samadhi the whole day.

Meditation, prayer and contemplation will lead you to meditation in action. Remember, you are a beloved child of the Lord. One way of liberation is to serve others and do your actions lovingly, skillfully and without any attachment. Speak lovingly, so you do not hurt or harm anyone. Try to be constantly aware of the truth. If somebody commits a mistake against you, you should forgive them. You should be able to forgive others, but first you should learn to forgive yourself. In addition, you should regularly exercise and do deep breathing exercises three times a day and regulate your eating and sleeping habits. It can be dangerous to be lost in the external world, but if you are lost within yourself, sooner or later you will have to find a way through love and meditation. Express love in your external life through your speech and actions.

Meditation in silence should lead you to meditation in action during the day. A systematic practice of meditation will prepare you for meditation in action. The finest part of meditation is to apply meditation in your daily actions, so that you are performing your actions while doing meditation. A human being cannot live without doing their duties. They have to act. But they can become lost when they do something. So that you are not lost, if you maintain your center and remember your mantra while doing your duties, that is meditation in action. Enjoy whatever you do in your daily life. Don't do what you do not enjoy.

Outside Indian villages there are plazas where the village wells are located. These plazas provide a safe environment for women. The women of the village go to those plazas with a small vessel on the top of the head to collect water from those wells. Having collected the water they place the vessel on their head and with all their vanity and pride they walk, dance and sing, and even sometimes cry, but the vessel doesn't fall. This is called meditation in action. If you do your duties no matter where you go, whatever you do and remember the Lord is seated deep within, that is meditation in action. No matter what happens, wherever you are, be aware of the reality within. That is the way of reaching the other shore of life.

the TECHNIQUE of MEDITATION

GENERAL ADVICE

Now, I want to give you instructions in how to meditate systematically. Patanjali has recommended a definite and very scientific method of meditation. Unfortunately, there is much misunderstanding about the nature of meditation. There are no tricks to learn for meditation. The process of meditation has to be systematically studied from both the scientific and the intuitive points of view. You cannot skip any of the steps. If from the very beginning you systematically follow the path, then it is not difficult. There are two ways to undertake the practice of meditation: the first way is to practise, then to experience and realize; the other way is to first understand the whole method of meditation and then practise. Both ways can be used.

ENVIRONMENT

Certain favorable conditions are required in the early stages of meditation. First, you should meditate in a clean, quiet and pleasant environment where you will not be disturbed.

My master was very practical. He said, "You know, we have appointed one old sadhu to sit outside the cave. He knows nothing about the scriptures and has not done any austerities. I told him to grow a big beard and look nice, so anyone who comes and touches his feet, he blesses outside. In this way, those inside are spared."

So, everybody thought he was a man of wisdom, but actually he was not very intelligent. We used to pay him to do this. I asked my master, "Is this not deception?"

He agreed that it was. I said, "Is it not sin?"

He said, "No."

I said, "Why not?"

He said, "To protect the flowers that are blooming inside the garden, you have to have a hedge that has thorns. We are grateful to him because he protects us and he gets money. People come and bow in front of him and he says, 'God bless you.'"

TEMPERATURE: It must be remembered that mind can only work well within certain limits of temperature. The greatest mental activity and mental efficiency is said to be around a temperature of 78 degrees F, and the greatest body efficiency is at the temperature of 68 degrees.

FOOD: The mind cannot work when the stomach is filled with food or when the bloodstream is surcharged with ingested food essence. Food makes the breath more vigorous and the mind in turn becomes more restless. Two meals a day is the best plan in the beginning, nothing but water or a small portion of milk to be taken in the intervals.

TIME: It is helpful to meditate at a fixed time each day. One can experiment for a few days until a definite time for daily practice is established. In the beginning don't make yourself sit for a long time because your body is not accustomed to remain without movement, and your posture will become distorted. Overdoing one's practice is certain to bring about mental dullness and tiredness, preventing true progress. Always be moderate in your habits and practice. If you spend ten minutes a day for one month just sitting quietly you will come to know many things about yourself. Many of you sit for a long time thinking that which you could not do in half an hour's time, perhaps you could do it in two and a half hours' time. Don't do that. You will only be wasting your time and energy. It is also not good to sit for meditation when you are very tired or you have eaten too much. Many of you sit down and immediately sleep comes. It is better not to meditate if you are tired, because your mind will slip to the valley of sleep. When your mind is tired and you start to lose awareness or feel sleepy, or you just start to day dream, you should not force yourself to sit for meditation. For the sake of experiment, for one week sit at exactly the same time and for not more than ten or fifteen minutes. But that time should be intense training. If an adept were to meditate for ten or eleven minutes, they would be in samadhi.

PREPARATION FOR MEDITATION

If you want to practise meditation, you have to slowly prepare yourself by cultivating an attitude of readiness for meditation. You should work with your body first, not because your body is something great that can lead you to meet God or to experience samadhi, but because it can be a great obstacle if you do not understand it. The body should be healthy and free from disease. It is helpful to perform preliminary exercises for cleansing the nervous system and regulating the motion of the lungs. Otherwise, the body can become a source of pain and misery for you. If the body is not kept healthy, then the mind will be constantly distracted. This is why the first step is to learn to work with your body. The body is a very useful instrument but it can become a barrier on the path of meditation.

In addition, a mind that has not been prepared systematically will refuse to cooperate. You may think you are already perfect so you can straight away meditate, but if you are not fully prepared, you will not be able to attain anything. You have to prepare yourself for meditation by deciding with firm conviction that at such and such time you will meditate, no matter what happens: *Nothing is going to interfere with my meditation. When my meditation time comes – I am Lord!* There was one blind man who used to sing a poem: *I am a king when I sing, though I am a poor blind boy.* Likewise, I am a king when I am in meditation. I could not sacrifice that moment even if God were to tell me to stop because I have practised my whole life. Even the greatest of siddhas never stop meditating, because that's what they have done for many lifetimes.

To do meditation you need to understand two things—*vairagya* (non-attachment) and *abhyasa* (practice). *Abhyasa vairagyabhyam tan nirodha.* With the help of constant practice and nonattachment you can have control over your mind and its modifications. Abhyasa and vairagya are the two wings of the bird that has decided to cross the mire of delusion. Non-attachment without practice is not complete. Non-attachment does not mean that you should not enjoy all the things of the world. All the things of the world have been given to you to enjoy, but you have to remember they are not yours, so you should not get attached to them. The best things in the world should be enjoyed and can be enjoyed, but remember that NOTHING IN THE WORLD CAN GIVE YOU HAPPINESS. You should use the things of the world as a means, but you should not be attached to them because you are not the proprietor. LET GO OF WHAT YOU ARE CLINGING TO AND YOU WILL HAVE WHAT YOU NEED. Without non-attachment one cannot lead the path of light. If you can strengthen this attitude within, you will be there. The philosophy of non-attachment means love.

You should prepare yourself for meditation by learning two things: how to be STILL and how to pay ATTENTION to what you are doing. For a few minutes every day you should learn to sit still, make your breath serene and your mind calm. Practice will make you perfect, not theory. No one can meditate for you. A guru, teacher or priest can give you blessings, but you have to practise meditation yourself. Buddha clearly said, "YOU HAVE TO LIGHT THY OWN LAMP. Nobody can give you salvation." You will have to meditate for yourself. You do your individual karmas, you have your individual mind and emotions and you know yourself better. You have to establish a state of tranquillity and peace. For a few minutes you should be completely away from body consciousness and consciousness of the world. Those moments are very good for health and will increase the longevity of your life.

Don't expect too much from yourself. That will only create guilt feelings within you. And don't try to jump suddenly to a higher level. You should have a regular, systematic schedule of practice. Go slowly and gently with yourself. Good students learn meditation systematically: how to sit still in a particular posture, keeping the head, neck, and trunk straight; how to breathe harmoniously by using diaphragmatic motion; then, how to create a joyous atmosphere that is conducive to meditation. From the very beginning, stillness and meditation should give you joy.

STEP BY STEP

There are different stages in the process of learning to meditate. You should practise and master them gradually, preferably under the guidance of a competent teacher. First are posture and body awareness, then breath awareness, mind and soul. To begin the process of meditation, sit down quietly and surrender your small self. When you practise yoga you become more aware, and body awareness leads you within to awareness of prana. Then, you become aware of the thinking process and you become more sensitive to the unconscious. The unconscious is a vast part of mind that is sleeping because you do not know how to use it. When you increase your capacity you can start to make more use of it. In addition, you become aware of the functions of the sympathetic and the parasympathetic systems.

MEDITATIVE POSTURE

First, ask yourself to be still and not to move. To gain mastery over one's self the student should sit firmly and still in a meditative posture, avoiding external disturbances of light, noise and changes of temperature. A comfortable and steady pose eliminates physical disturbances and frees the mind for the efforts of concentration. You do not know how much joy and clarity of mind you can derive when you sit quietly.

So, the first step is to sit in a COMFORTABLE, STEADY and STILL posture. The greatest of all strength comes from stillness and inner silence. According to yoga, you cannot be still if you do not know certain rules. If you learn to be still, you can come to enjoy that peace that cannot be provided by any object in the world and you can experience something great and profound, something that you could never have even imagined previously. This is explained by Sutra 1:46 that describes the proper posture for meditation: *Sthira sukham asanam. Asanam* refers to posture, *sthira* means "steadiness," and *sukham* means "comfortable." People often ask which meditative posture they should choose: the lotus posture, the accomplished pose or the easy pose. As long as the spinal column is correctly aligned, you can choose any posture you want. Choose a posture that is both steady and comfortable, not one that is steady but creates pain for you. Steadiness of posture, according to the science of meditation means to keep your head, neck and trunk aligned, and assimilate your upper and lower extremities into a comfortable and correct posture. If you are sitting with your legs correctly in padmasana but your head is not straight and your neck is bending, then it is not padmasana.

Many people have strange ideas about meditative postures. They think that good posture means twisting their legs and making their form elegant. Meditation has nothing to do with the upper and lower extremities, except that they should be arranged so that the spinal column remains comfortably aligned. You should be steady and at the same time comfortable no matter how you arrange your upper extremities and lower extremities. The spine is the center of the yogic body. The arms and legs might disturb and distort your position and create stress on your posture. Assimilate your limbs in such as a way that they don't disturb the body and your spinal column remains aligned. You can sit comfortably on the edge of a straight-back chair, as long as your head, neck and trunk are straight. That is also a meditative posture, *maitri asana*, the friendship posture. Remember that if you sit correctly for ten minutes a day for fifteen days, you will attain some progress.

When my master asked me how long I could sit in one posture, I replied, "One hour 45 minutes."

Then, he instructed me to bring his cane to him. I knew something was definitely going to happen. He put the cane by his side as he sat down and told me to sit down with him. He didn't use his cane, but that was the first time I was able to sit for five hours because of the fear of the cane. If you don't have any fear what will happen?

BODY AWARENESS

To study your body you need to pay attention to it. You can study the body once you have learned to make your body still. When you start to practise how to sit, you will notice your body cannot remain still for very long. Even though you apply a posture to create stillness you find that you are not still. Your body keeps moving and remains restless. Initially, these gross movements are disturbing. After a few days, you will find that they will have stopped, but then you may notice subtle twitching that can create other problems for you. When the muscles or any part of the body throbs or twitches, that is not a sign of progress; it is just the release of tension. Even if it takes two to six months to attain a steady, comfortable posture, once you can sit quietly, the next step comes.

Now, first be aware of the body and put a question: *Who am I? Am I the body? No. I have a body, but I am not the body. I am also a breathing, sensing and thinking being.* You think you are body alone because you have not been made aware of anything further. All these feelings and thoughts are called superimpositions. They are good teachings to help you live in the world and communicate with others, but they do not lead you to the higher dimensions.

Observe your body to see if there is tension. If you find there is tension, you have to find out the cause from the four fountains: food, sleep, sex and self-preservation. You become stressed when you eat bad food because food affects the mind. You cannot sleep if your mind is disturbed and you feel stressed when you are overdoing sex. When you start to question and analyze, finally you realize that you have an urge that is called self-preservation. All fears come from self-preservation. You needlessly feel afraid all the time. When you are insecure, you are afraid. Fear means you are afraid you might lose something, you might die or you might not gain what you want. You want to protect yourself because of the sense of self-preservation and because you do not understand your relationship with the ultimate reality. However, the sense of self-protection is not found on all levels. You are not concerned about protecting the divinity in you. You just want to protect your physical self because you think it is the instrument that will help you fulfill the purpose of life. You have to regulate these four fountains of the emotions.

BREATH AWARENESS

Even if you can still the body, you do not know how to deal with the breath yet. So, the next step is to focus your mind on your breath so that mind and breath become perfectly coordinated. Breath and mind are twin laws of life that function together. Even if you just think negatively, the breath will change dramatically and the motion of the lungs will be disturbed. This will affect the whole body. You should take one or two months' time to work on the breath. Sixty per cent of the distraction of the mind is created by bad breathing habits. Also, irregularities or excesses in the four urges of food, sex, sleep and desire for self-preservation can negatively change your breathing pattern.

Breath awareness is very interesting. Let your mind pay attention toward the breath and allow your mind to flow with the breath. With your mind locate the point from where the breath starts to come back toward you. After that just rest in the one-pointed mind for a few minutes. This is difficult to attain and it will take some time. Just ask your mind to feel the air passing through the nostrils. Both nostrils are flowing freely and you are inhaling and exhaling from both nostrils. With the practice of breath awareness the mind gradually calms down. You can become aware there is one center from where the vital energy is being supplied, and there is another center within you where you are receiving it. On one line there are only two ends, so there is no difference between you and the reality. You are always in harmony with the reality. Direct experience will lead you to this state of mind.

HOW TO BREATHE

The breath can disturb you in many ways, but it can be controlled very easily. To overcome disturbances of the breath, you should regulate exhalation and inhalation so they are of the same length. Regulated breath helps to strengthen the nervous system and calm the mind. Once you have done so, you can meditate on the breath. Meditation on the breath means to be aware that you are breathing and how you are breathing. Your breath naturally becomes finer when you become still. Breath and mind become integrated so that you may have the feeling you are not breathing. This is an encouraging sign that you are advancing.

You should simply observe a few things about your breathing habits. The breath should be smooth without jerks and silent without the noise that comes from blocked nostrils. In addition, it should be deep and relaxed and without any useless pauses. You have to make your breath serene so the motion of the lungs does not disturb you. When the breathing becomes irregular it disturbs the autonomic nervous system so the exchange of oxygen and carbon dioxide becomes imbalanced and it becomes difficult to remain steady in meditation. It might take several months to learn to regulate the breath.

Next, mind observes that while you are exhaling and inhaling you are unconsciously creating a pause. The moment you create a pause, it disturbs your heart and the right vagus nerve. When the right vagus nerve is disturbed, the motion of the lungs is disturbed and the pumping motion of the heart to your brain is interrupted. Your memory will also be affected. A long pause means death. If you inhale and never exhale you will die. Similarly, if you exhale and never inhale you will die. Those animals that breathe shallowly do not live for a long time. But if you practise inhalation and exhalation without any pause, you will find mind becomes very calm instead of jumping here and there. When you learn to gradually control the pause, the inhalation and exhalation becomes like an unbroken wave arising and merging. If you can eliminate the pause between inhalation and exhalation, then you also have the power to expand the pause. I am not teaching you something injurious. Your body will tell you when to stop so you don't go beyond your capacity. When you become too breathless, a point will come when your body will start to shake along with perspiration because you are straining. If you do not accept something you experience mental strain, and that mental strain leads to strain and agitation in the nervous system. After a few days of practice you will observe that you are able to arrest unwanted body movements.

In the ancient scriptures the science of breath is called *prana vedana*. Yogis live according to the number of breaths they take. Thus, you can expand your life expectancy if you understand this practical science that is known to only a fortunate few. Those who know this science can suspend their breath for a long time, even for months at a time. But as a beginner you will not have to go so deep. The particular group that practises this is called *pranavedin* — those who know the mysteries of the pranas, the subtler forces of life. Your usual way of breathing is to exhale, then pause; then you inhale, and a pause comes. So you should try to omit those two pauses. You also have the capacity to expand to hold the pause. That is called *kumbhaka*. Exhalation is *rechaka;* inhalation is *puraka.* Don't jump here and there or try to practise kumbhaka (retention) immediately. Just practise how to omit the pause, because PAUSE MEANS DEATH. In the beginning, breathing exercises are meant to regulate the motion of lungs. Finally, all the breathing and pranayama exercises are meant to help you to have perfect control over the pause. These techniques are not so secret. The teacher imparts them to those students that are prepared, and are sincerely practising.

Breath is like a barometer that registers both your mental and physical conditions. The study of the breath is a science in itself. In the modern world, not much research has been done on the breath, but yogis have done extensive research. There is only one proprietor who is supplying the life breath to all of us. BREATH IS LIFE AND LIFE IS BREATH.

BREATHING EXERCISES

Breathing exercises are therapeutic. Breath and mind coordination can help you to alleviate many mental and nervous disorders. Breathing exercises are meant to regulate inhalation and exhalation, the two guards of the city of life. Let your mind flow with the flow of your breath. The moment you think you are breathing, what will happen to you? You will take a deep breath. It means awareness leads you toward fulfillment.

DIAPHRAGMATIC BREATHING

There is a difference between yogic breathing and normal breathing. The highest of all breathing techniques is diaphragmatic breathing. Now, you have to learn to breathe diaphragmatically and regulate the breath so it becomes calm, serene and deep. The diaphragm is a dome-shaped muscle located beneath the lungs. When you exhale, the upper abdomen should push into help the diaphragm contract and push against the lungs to expel the carbon dioxide. When you inhale, the upper abdomen should spontaneously relax so the diaphragm can release to allow the lungs to make more space for oxygen. One inhales by contracting the diaphragm. This downward pressure forces the upper abdomen outward and sucks air into the lungs. This should become your habitual way of breathing. You should practise for five minutes three times a day. The capacity of the diaphragmatic muscle is tremendous, but it takes practice to make the diaphragm stronger. You can use sand bags or other weights up to 12 pounds to do that. By properly regulating the movement of the diaphragm one can induce a profound physical relaxation and calmness, cooling down an overcharged body or turning off internal stress responses.

Many of you are committing a mistake thinking that you are doing diaphragmatic breathing, but you are actually doing abdominal breathing and calling it diaphragmatic breathing. There is a difference. The lower abdomen should remain relaxed as it is not involved in diaphragmatic breathing. Diaphragmatic breathing can help you to prevent many diseases. It's very good for the heart and the lungs.

NADI SHODANAM

Pay attention to the flow of breath through the two nostrils. After a few days, you will notice when one nostril is prominently active, the other becomes passive. Then after some time, a switch takes place and the active nostril becomes passive, while the passive nostril is now active. Also, breathing through the left nostril is different from breathing through the right. Air flowing through the left nostril will signal restfulness and calm such as in sleep, while when the right nostril breathing predominates, the body is prepared for more active processes such as are needed in digestion. The nostrils should be cleaned regularly by pouring lukewarm, saline water first through one nostril and then through the other, allowing it to flow out of the opposite side.

Once you have established a calm even rhythm to your breathing, you can practise nadi shodanam, alternate nostril breathing, using the thumb and middle finger of the right hand to alternately close and open each nostril to regulate the flow of the breath. After some time, you should be able to regulate the flow of the breath through alternate nostrils with the mind, for mind and breath are very close friends and are dependent on each other.

RELAXATION

The next step is to relax. Many of you do not actually understand the meaning of relaxation. To relax does not mean to go to sleep. One can be completely relaxed if one knows how to breathe correctly, because proper breathing helps to release stress and strain on all levels — body, nervous system and mind. You cannot become relaxed merely by loosening the muscles. In many clinics all over the world people say *relax, relax, relax* and tell you to loosen the muscles. That is not relaxation. There are two methods of relaxation, ancient and modern. The ancient method is scientific and systematic; the modern one is suggestive. If you tell someone to lie down and say *relax, relax,* such suggestions do not work. Instead, you should lead people toward self-awareness in such a way so there is no suggestion in it. *Relaxation* means "to have perfect control over the contraction and relaxation of your muscles." When you want to contract or relax your muscles, you should be able to do that. This requires control over the autonomic or involuntary nervous system. Any other relaxation is false.

BREATHING AND RELAXATION PRACTICUM

Lie in savasana. Don't allow your mind to roam around, but gently focus the mind within. First, pay attention to the flow of your breath. Take five deep, even breaths, without creating any noise, jerks or pause in the breath. Observe the movement of the upper abdomen with the breath. Now, shift the focus of the mind from the breath to the body. Be aware of your toes. From the tips of the toes systematically release any tension from your toes, feet, ankles, knees, hip joints, perineum, abdomen, chest, hands, forearms, upper arms, chest, neck and face. Allow the whole body to release all tension. When you exhale the breath, exhale all tension and worries from the mind. Now exhale slowly as though you are exhaling from the crown of your head to your toes. Then again inhale the energy from the toes back to the crown of your head. On the next exhalation, exhale to the ankles and inhale from the ankles back to the crown of your head. Exhale to your knees and inhale from the knees to the crown of your head. Exhale to the perineum, and inhale from the perineum to the crown of your head. Exhale to the navel and inhale from the navel to the crown of your head. Exhale to the space between the two breasts and inhale up to the crown of your head. Exhale to your throat center and inhale to the crown of your head. Now, exhale to the bridge between the two nostrils. This is very important. Let your mind focus on the place between the two nostrils, asking your mind to allow the breath to flow freely through both nostrils. Follow the flow of breath between the bridge between the two nostrils and the crown of your head. You will find the breath has become very fine. Now, relax and exhale from the crown of your head down to the throat center. Breathe deeply from the throat center to the crown of your head, exhaling down to the heart center. Again inhale to the crown of your head. Then exhale to the navel center, inhaling back to the crown of your head. Exhale to the perineum, and come back to the crown of your head. Exhale to the knees, again come back to the crown of your head. Exhale to the ankles, inhale coming back to the crown of your head. Exhale to your toes, inhale from your toes to the crown of your head. Now let your whole body exhale and inhale. The movement of the breath is like a wave in the ocean. Inhalation is like a wave rising from the ocean; exhalation is like a wave going back to the ocean. Remember the body is your grossest instrument, the breath is a subtler instrument and even subtler are the senses. The mind is your subtlest instrument. When you regulate the breath, you are actually training your mind. But you are not body, breath, senses and mind. Your essential nature is peace, happiness and wisdom. Now breathe gently to your fullest capacity.

CONTROL OF PRANA

In the third stage of meditation one learns the control of prana—the vital energy behind all your breathing, thoughts and actions. The lungs can function with a minimum amount of oxygen. Prana is much more than oxygen. It is described as a current of energy. There are special nerve centers (chakras) in the body that when aroused can give you complete control over your body. For this, you should learn the science of prana. It is only through meditation and yogic breathing that one gains control over inhalation and exhalation and thus subsequently can become master of their prana.

PRATYAHARA

You have to adjust yourself so that the external world does not create barriers and problems for you. Otherwise, whenever you sit you will find that the images and thoughts of whatever is happening to you in the external world will dominate your meditation. Once you have made your breath calm, you will have to practise pratyahara, to become aware of the reality. When consciousness is turned within in the intermediate step of pratyahara, your awareness may have withdrawn from external objects, but still you are aware of your own shape and form. In order to disconnect the conscious mind from the senses, mind has to remain pleasantly busy. Conscious withdrawal of the mind from the senses does not mean that you have to withdraw from life and its purpose. It can be done with the help of breath control and mind control. Once you have withdrawn your senses, nothing will disturb you from outside because you are no longer seeing, tasting, smelling, touching or listening.

However, the moment you close your eyes, you are immediately faced with the day to day problems that you are storing and have stored before. If you go a little bit deeper, then your childhood problems will come up. Also, all your planning, postponements and engagements come forward during that time. That's what you do and you call it meditation.

Meditation is an entirely new venture for your mind, so it will be a little bit difficult. The mind does not want to meditate because you have formed some bad habits. It is better to attend to your breath before you do meditation. You can temporarily control your mind by having control over the breath because it is related to the mind. And then, let your breath flow freely and follow your mind. So far, mind runs very easily with the help of the senses to the external world. Now, you have to guide mind toward the unknown without any images, forms or names. When you try to become an insider, suddenly you come in touch with your mental life, your thought forms and internal states. But when you are all alone you have to understand who you are and what you want to do with your life. Then you know that you have to deal with your mind. When you have learned to breathe in a calm and serene way, then you go to the next step. Mind should be kept free from all intruding thoughts. The breath will then gradually become steadier and steadiness of the mind will follow. With regular practice night and day, the breathing comes under control and as the practice progresses the mind becomes calm and steady.

SUSHUMNA

I have explained to you the fundamentals of meditation—the value of a posture that is still, steady and comfortable and the value of regulated breathing. Your breath patterns and your brain wave patterns are completely controlled by your thinking process. If mind is not in a healthy state, you cannot regulate the breath. If you really want to advance in meditation, you will have to practise three advanced techniques: First, apply sushumna and then sushumna awakening—awakening the power that you have within. Then, you have to learn how to direct and use that power. When you close your eyes and become quiet, you become aware you have a body. Your body is moved by a certain power that exists within as a reservoir of energy. There are many names for that energy depending on which level you have reached:

primal force, spiritual energy, kundalini, dormant power and psychic energy, to name a few.

THREE MAIN NADIS: There are three main nadis (energy channels) closely associated with the three physical cords located along the spinal column. The cords originate at the base of the spine and the nadis arise from the lowest chakra, muladhara, where the serpent energy kundalini lies intoxicated. The three physical cords are the centralis canalis in the center of the spine and the two ganglionated cords (sympathetic and parasympathetic) that run along the sides of the spinal cord upward to be connected to the medulla oblongata. The medulla oblongata is related to your autonomic nervous system and the control of your entire physical life and also a part of your mind. That particular part of mind that is being controlled by your autonomic nervous system should be brought under control first.

The nadis represent the energy forces that flow along the pathways of ida, pingala and sushumna. The centralis canalis corresponds to the more subtle and very important nadi through which the energy of sushumna flows. Likewise, the two ganglionated cords correspond to the subtle nadis ida (parasympathetic) and pingala (sympathetic). Just as electricity is different from the wires it traverses, the subtle forces that flow through the nadis are different from the nadis. On their journey upward, ida and pingala criss cross along the spine while passing through the chakras. The ida nadi terminates in the left nostril, and the pingala nadi in the right nostril. Sushumna nadi terminates in the space between the two eyebrows (ajna chakra) and then down to the bridge between the two nostrils.

Ida and pingala are the two basic energies of all human beings. Ida and the left nostril are associated with nourishing energy characterized as feminine in nature and cooling like the moon. It is intuitive, inward and passive. On the other hand, pingala and the right nostril is active and more externally oriented. It is characterized as the male energy and is heating like the sun. As opposed to the inward nature of ida, pingala is more rational.

THE PRACTICE OF SUSHUMNA AWAKENING: As you are sitting in your meditative posture and have established a smooth, even rhythm to your diaphragmatic breath, move your awareness to the flow of breath in the two nostrils. Notice which nostril is more open and active; focus on the active nostril for a few breaths and then move your awareness to the passive nostril. As you do this, you will notice the passive nostril becomes open and active. After a few breaths, shift your attention to the bridge between the two nostrils and feel the two breaths unite in a single stream. Inhale from the bridge between the nostrils up to the center of ajna chakra, and then exhale back to the bridge between the nostrils. Mentally listen to the sound *soooo* as you inhale, and as you exhale follow the sound *hummmmmmm.* Concentration on this movement of the central breath will create a joyous state of mind, conducive to meditation.

NOSTRIL PREDOMINANCE: As described previously in the discussion of nadi shodanam, whenever you are inhaling and exhaling, you will notice one of the nostrils remains open and predominant, while the other remains closed or blocked. The nostril that seems to be blocked is passive. The moment you pay attention to the passive nostril, it will open and become active. This situation continues for some time, and then they alternate so the open nostril closes and the closed nostril opens. They continue to alternate in regular intervals throughout the day. During the brief space of time while the predominant nostril is changing to the other nostril, you will experience a state of harmony in which you are inhaling and exhaling through both nostrils. It is a very small moment but very joyous. You can expand that moment of joy by practising the application of sushumna.

SUSHUMNA APPLICATION: When both nostrils flow freely, that is a sign and symptom of the application of sushumna. This will happen when you focus on the bridge between the two nostrils. By applying sushumna, you are preparing your mind to meditate by creating a joyous condition for your mind. In order to meditate you should have a joyous mind, no matter what is happening in the external world. You are joyous by nature but you have created many problems for yourself, so your joy has changed into pain.

With the application of sushumna, you can consciously cut off with the external world, check the usual habits of the mind and make your mind very joyous so that mind no longer suffers pain, distractions or dissipations. If you apply sushumna, your body will no longer be a source of distraction to you. It will feel very light and comfortable and you will feel as though you are going higher and higher. This means your mind is detached from your body consciousness and is trying to fathom inwardness. For a few days you might experience difficulty because you have never trained yourself. But if you can do it, it will be hard to believe the joy you will have. I can guarantee that nothing in the world could ever give you such joy. Even when I am busy and doing my work, I feel that joy. Even if I am scolding somebody, inside my heart I feel joy. Nothing in the world could ever give you that particular joy. Be joyous and conduct your work accordingly. Sushumna awakening is very important. If you cannot apply sushumna to allow both nostrils to flow freely, it means your mind is disorderly and you are not ready for meditation.

SANDHYA: The particular moment when both nostrils are flowing freely is referred to as the wedding of your right nostril and your left nostril, or the sun is wedding the moon. This is called sandhya. What a great joy there will be when the two are wedded. If you apply sushumna, the focus of your mind will immediately go to the sushumna channel where it connects to the reservoir of the dormant force to awaken that force. So the application of sushumna and the awakening of sushumna are very important for meditation.

KUNDALINI AWAKENING: Then comes kundalini awakening. When you apply sushumna, you are going to the interior world, where there is a vast reservoir of dormant energy. You have to know how to handle that energy. Kundalini awakening is not what you think it is. It means to fathom the many levels of consciousness. If you have not awakened that energy, your capacity will remain limited. But when you have awakened the energy you will be able to do and see everything. If you slowly increase your capacity you will gain more and more knowledge until finally you become one with the absolute reality and you are free.

MIND and MEDITATION

STUDY of MIND
CONDITIONINGS of MIND
CATEGORIES of MIND
FUNCTIONS of MIND
INNER DIALOGUE
CONSCIOUS and UNCONSCIOUS
MIND CONTROL
TRAIN of THOUGHTS
BE STILL and KNOW
OBSTACLES to MEDITATION
SENSATIONS
LETTING GO
WITNESSING
INTROSPECTION
TYPES of THOUGHT PATTERNS
INNER LIGHT and SOUNDS
MIND POWER
MEDITATION PRACTICUMS

STUDY OF MIND

Once you have learned to be still and can control your breathing, you can start to work with your mind. Mind is your finest instrument. As the breath gradually becomes steadier, steadiness of the mind will follow. When you try to understand your mind you will come to know mind is a great magician. As you sit and observe the workings of your mind, mind will unfold itself before you and you will find out how it plays tricks and how powerful it is. There are so many dimensions of the mind that no matter how much you think you understand your mind there is always something more to know. There are many modifications of your mind and various levels: personal mind, transpersonal mind, inner mind, collective mind and cosmic mind. It will take a long time, but with the help of samyama (concentration, meditation and samadhi) you can come to understand all the levels of your mind.

It is your mind that stands between you and the reality, because mind habitually identifies with external objects that keep you from becoming aware of your essential nature. This is why you remain in a state of confusion. In that state, you have conflicts within and without and you don't know what to do. You identify with the objects of the world instead of remembering the reality within. You are wasting your time, energy and intelligence. You have to practise meditation in order to purify your mind so that your mind does not come in your way. If you purify your mind, it will not create obstacles and you will be free. YOU HAVE TO GO BEYOND YOUR MIND to become aware of the reality.

The mind is a train of thoughts, emotions, desires, motivations and ambitions. You can't make a single gesture without the help of your mind. Your body is only a garment and is very small compared to the mind. THE WHOLE OF THE BODY IS IN THE MIND, BUT THE WHOLE OF THE MIND IS NOT IN THE BODY. Your prayers, good actions, writings, thoughts and speech are all subject to your mind. Mind constantly jumps; wherever you go, it is not there. You should understand how mind functions and you should be very practical when you study your mind. You have every right to understand your mind.

According to Eastern psychology, you have to study mind from various angles. Mind is studied by its patterns, its thinking process and by analyzing and categorizing certain emotions. When you find out you have had many failures and have made many mistakes you don't know how to deal with all that. Once you have understood your mind in its entirety with all its faculties, then you would have known what is to be known. And when you come in touch with the many different levels of your mind, you will be able to serve, love and understand others better. There is no need to go to a fortune teller, psychic or a swami to know your mind. Self-dependency will give you self-confidence. No doubt you need a teacher to guide you. I would never tell you not to study books or learn from other people. I have met people who were not educated and did not know anything. Whenever we had any difficulty we would approach them, and they alone were able to give us a solution. Sometimes you consult a priest or a swami, or other persons you think could be helpful to you, but you neglect to go to the great guru that is seated within you. LOOK WITHIN, FIND WITHIN. How to find and how to look within? Pray.

CONDITIONINGS OF MIND

No matter how much you concentrate your mind or how much you meditate and contemplate, it's not going to help if you have not understood the conditionings of the mind: TIME, SPACE and CAUSATION. You should understand and systematically deal with the prime conditionings of your mind, because they are very important. Without understanding these conditionings, you may be able to have a concentrated mind and make your mind one-pointed and inward but still you will not have mental freedom from those conditionings. Because your mind is conditioned by time, space and causation, before you make any commitment to undertake the practice of meditation you want to know how long it is going to take. It is more appropriate to ask yourself if you have time and if you can discipline yourself to meditate every day punctually and regularly. You cannot expand your consciousness if you don't practise regularly. Reluctantly, you answer you can spare some time, but only if you are assured of gaining something. In meditation, you should have only one thought for a prolonged time. If there are two thoughts, then the conditions of time, space and causation will be there; but if there is only one thought there will be no conditions. As long as mind is conditioned by time it is not meditation. You may be making effort to meditate, but you have not yet attained it. Time, space and causation are three conditions of mind that have created maya (ignorance).

TIME: PAST, PRESENT AND FUTURE: All minds are conditioned by time, the biggest filter there is. You should learn to go beyond time by studying how mind is conditioned by time. Suppose you are sad today and very worried. You may even be thinking of committing suicide. After going through the natural filter of time, the next day you may no longer want to commit suicide.

There is a very fine line between the three main conditionings of time: past, present and future. Only with the help of meditation and samyama can you get freedom from these conditionings. And when you get freedom, your mind will have the power to know your past and future because your mind will have gone beyond the bounds of time, space and causation.

When the kundalini shakti awakens, you will be better able to understand time, space and causation. Past, present and future will be nothing to you because you will have gone beyond the ordinary mind. Time is created by the mind, and time and mind are closely related. Many thoughts are coming and you call it the thinking process. A thought comes, followed by another thought and then again another thought. There is a space between every two thoughts. Japa is done to eliminate the space between two thoughts. If there is no space between two thoughts, there will also be no time or causation. Similarly, if there is only one thought there will be no space at all. This means there is only One. That is why when you are constantly aware of the truth there is no space between your thoughts. But if there is no space between two thoughts then what will happen to time? Time will not exist. So time and space are variations of the same thing. If there is only one thought in the mind, time will have no effect. Many thoughts will come and go, but beneath all those thoughts there is only one consciousness. You can become free only when you have profound knowledge of the one absolute without second. Such a mind has the power to penetrate into the deeper levels of your being.

IF NOT NOW, WHEN? If you know two words, you have known everything: SILENCE and NOW. You should remember that a human being is a nucleus and the universe is its expansion. There would be no sense of the universe without human beings. A human being is an evolved being, though unfinished, but desiring to attain perfection. You can do that if you learn how not to be obsessed by the past or by the fear and imagination of the future. You talk about here and *now* but you do not understand what the present is. The moment you talk of the present, the present has gone to the past. So actually, there is nothing like the present at all. Anything that you think of suddenly slips to the past. And then, on the basis of the memory of the past, you think of the future. Whatever you are today, it is just your past. You do not know what *now* means, how to attain *now*, how to be in the *now* or how to live in the *now*. You can spell the word *now*, but you do not know what it is. BE HERE AND NOW AND YOU WILL BE FREE. If you can get freedom from past experiences and you can stop your mind from imagining the future, you will enjoy *now*. There is no other way if you do not meditate. I am not talking about the Indian way or the Buddhist way of meditation. I am talking about the way that can help you to enjoy here and *now*. If you do not live in the silence and in the now, you are here but you remain scattered. Make effort to put yourself into silence sometimes. A real human being is one who knows how to live here and *now*. Only when mind is free from past memories and imagination of the future can mind be brought to a state of *now*. You think the objects of the world have the power to give you enjoyment. That is not true. No object has the power to give you enjoyment. Enjoyment comes when you learn how to be here and *now*. This is possible when you make your mind free from all conditionings and then try to be still.

PAST AND FUTURE: Those who know how to link past and future by knowing *now* can go beyond time, space and causation. That which is going to happen after six months, they can know right *now*. This does not mean they are controlling their destiny; they just know what they are going to do. When you have gone beyond time, you can know what you are going to do day after tomorrow without any predetermination. The person who is on top of the mountain can see what is going on behind the mountain and below the mountain all the time. This does not mean anything is predetermined. If you believe in predetermination, then you will not do anything and you will be just become lazy. In the meantime, that which was going to happen will happen. You should use the method of meditation to live here and *now,* and then you will understand what is past and future.

If you slowly expand your field of consciousness, then you will be able to recall all of your past. First, you have to learn how to be still and to make your breath serene. Once you have made your breath calm you withdraw your senses. When you try to calm down the conscious mind, suddenly the unconscious mind becomes active and a rush of thoughts comes from the unconscious. Pleasant and unpleasant thought patterns will come. You have to know how to deal with those thought patterns and go beyond them. *This is not me, this is only my thought. Why should I get involved mentally when a thought is going through my mind?* You have to strengthen your sankalpa shakti and decide that mind is yours and you will not allow your mind to run here and there. In addition, you have to learn to witness your thoughts so you do not identify with them. If you can do this for a few minutes every day, you can change your thinking process.

You say this is all God's creation and you claim God has made you the way you are. This is not acceptable. Why would God, the Lord of equality, have such discrimination? If you are all at the mercy of God, then what good is meditation or doing good acts? If whatever you do is because of God's grace, it means you can never change or improve yourself. But the right philosophy says a human being is an unfinished being and has the opportunity to complete themself and attain wisdom in this lifetime. You can finally realize the highest summit of life, turiya. You can know about the future as much as you know about the past, because your future is totally dependent on your past memories. Patanjali is telling you that you have the power within to go beyond both past and future. However, Patanjali is talking only about those minds that have been properly trained so they have the power to go beyond to the source of memory and, on the basis of the past, can even go beyond the future. It can be done. You can train your mind to cross the line of the present and make your future and present one and the same. This doesn't mean that everything is pre-determined. Don't think that you cannot change anything. Your past is your own past, your present is your own present and your future is your own future. This is all your creation. So don't think you don't have the power to change your future. If you become aware that this is all your creation and it is time for you to change, you will be able to do so. Otherwise, there will be no future for you and you will be completely controlled by the past only. You have to be bold enough to face all the consequences of your past deeds. Even if the past was dark, you can utilize your present and make your future bright. If you change your course there is no need to be afraid the past will continue to affect you. It is important that you don't allow yourself to brood on the past. You postpone all joys and pleasures for the future, and that future never comes, but it remains as a sort of hope.

Those who claim to foretell the future can only prophesy what is going to happen; they cannot change anything. However, you have the power to change your destiny and expand your life. Then, those prophesies will not be realised. That is why even the prophesies of the scriptures do not always come true. You are the architect of your destiny. You can live for a long time if you know why and how. When I was seven years old, ten learned people of India said I was going to die at the age of 28 years. I am still here, and none of them are there. There is nothing like predestination, otherwise evolution and consciousness, knowledge and realization would have no sense. YOU HAVE TO DECIDE FOR YOURSELF. No one else decides for you.

There was one sage who was an expert who could tell people when they were going to die. He would tell people, "You can kill me if my prediction turns out to be wrong. You should arrange your affairs because you will die at such and such time on such and such date." However, when he met a yogi and he told him when he was going to die, the yogi said, "No. Death means separation and destruction of two vehicles—prana and apana—that are supplying life energy and cleansing the body. I will hide them where death has no access. Now, let me see if your predictions come true."

Even though that so-called expert predicted the yogi's death nine times, still the yogi did not die. If you know this science, death will be under your control. Death means destruction of the pranic vehicles. If you are a yogi and you know how to control these pranic vehicles, no predictions will ever come true. According to yoga science, death means not having control over your autonomic nervous system. That's why the body falls apart and one dies. It is possible to bring all these subtle functions under your control, by having control over your autonomic nervous system. There are two ways to do that. One is by having dynamic will power, and another is with the help of pranayama practices. A yogi can create death for themself any time they want if they know how to apply sushumna.

CATEGORIES OF MIND

Patanjali has described the levels of the mind in five categories: *kshipta, mudha, vikshipta, ekagra,* and *nirodha. Kshipta* is "a completely distracted mind." Those who are completely off are out of the question. Patanjali was aware of this particular category, but he did not start his science from that. He started with those who are normal. The mind that remains in a state of stupor is called *mudha. Vikshipta* applies to those who do not have a concentrated mind, but if they make effort, they can learn. Sometimes they understand and sometimes they do not because of their lack of attention. Their minds are not yet properly trained, but they are capable of being trained. *Ekagra* indicates the one-pointed mind that can concentrate well. *Nirodha* refers to the mind that is completely under control. *Nirodha parinama* is that transformation of the mind in which it becomes progressively permeated by the condition of nirodha. Such persons have perfectly trained their mind and can use it as they wish. For example, they can develop free will to any extent. But what is free will? I can stand on one leg. This is free will. However, I cannot stand without both legs. So, you have free will and you don't. But once you have control over mind, you can have complete free will and you can even float, if you want.

FUNCTIONS of MIND

One of the ways to understand mind is to study the various functions of mind. In Western psychology there is nothing like functions of mind. Education does not know how to train the totality of mind and the different functions of the mind. The body and the five *indriyas* (sight, hearing, smell, touch and taste) and the five *karmendriyas* (speech, ability to grasp, locomotion, excretion and procreation) are not sufficient to inspect the whole mind. Even the busiest people of this world do not use more than one-tenth of the mind. Modern psychiatry is not so advanced that it understands everything about mental life. Psychology and psychiatry do not properly know the nature of the mind so they do not know how to handle it. They are aware of the negative power of the mind, but they do not know how to awaken its positive power. The day they come to know the method of how to awaken the positive power of mind, they will find out that mind can also be used for healing purposes.

Patanjali has described in detail mind and its modifications, *chitta* and its *vrittis* and the various functions of the mind: MANAS (mind), CHITTA (storehouse of samskaras), BUDDHI (intellect), and AHANKARA (ego). Mind will try to confuse you by giving you many suggestions. Unless mind takes help from the buddhi, it will always be confused. Whenever you feel confused, it is because you have not properly consulted your buddhi.

If you do not understand your internal states, you will not be able to express yourself properly in the external world or communicate effectively with others. You don't need external help to understand your internal states; you just have to make your mind one-pointed. Then you will be able to understand all the faculties of mind, particularly the BUDDHI, the faculty of judgment. Everybody thinks they are intellectuals because they have the ability to think. In this context, *intellectual* means "mind keeps brooding on facts." Many couples cannot lead a peaceful life because they each have the habit of intellectualizing everything in the external world rather than trying to comprehend their emotional and feeling levels. The intellectual area is entirely different from the emotional area. So, first you will have to deal with that part of the intellect that broods without coming to any fruitful conclusion and is not capable of making decisions in time. You can easily train the buddhi if you learn a definite way of concentration. Once you have developed a decisive buddhi and have complete command over your mind and its modifications you will have reached the third stage. At this point you will be able to consciously tap into the unconscious reservoir of all your memories and experiences, past and present, and use them in your daily life. Great persons who know how to decide things in time are the most successful people in the world. This is true from a worldly point of view, and it is also true from a divine point of view. The key to all success lies in having developed your decisive faculty so that you can use it in your daily life.

Meditation can help you to understand all aspects of your mind and to train all the faculties and various functions of mind so that you can go beyond. Ordinarily, your mind works only within the small field of whatever you have seen, heard, thought of or imagined. The field of your mind is so small that mind is not able to help you. Mind is like a small scale and you are trying to measure the whole universe with the help of that small scale. This is not possible. Your limited mind tends to wander within a boundary of its own within the field of the phenomenal world, because you are not aware that it can go beyond to the state where mind is free from all forms and remains in a state of joy and happiness. Patanjali says you can cross that field, because there are many other fields. Now, you have to go beyond. *Beyond* means the "transpersonal field." Beyond does not mean far away or beyond reach; BEYOND MEANS WITHIN. You have to cross over to the transpersonal field where you will find that your mind is vast and open to receive new ideas. When you know the use of one function but do not know the use of the other functions of mind, you are not tapping the whole source. You should know the totality of yourself, something about body, nervous system, mind, transpersonal mind and the center of consciousness. Your conscious mind is beyond your senses, and your unconscious mind is beyond your conscious mind. Your transpersonal mind is beyond your mind, and Christ consciousness is beyond your transpersonal mind.

AHANKARA (ego) is also a prominent function of your mind. EGO CONTRACTS YOUR PERSONALITY. You have to face ego and use it as you use your shoes. You use your shoes so much they wear out. Another way to deal with ego is to use it in a creative way by leaving the lower dimensions and going to the higher dimensions of life. There are various ways to do that. Then, if ego comes forward during meditation, you will have to face it and deny it because ego does not allow you to understand transpersonal life or to go outside the field of your individual mind. There is no place for ego if you really want to be cheerful and happy. Ego has only one function and that is to help you conduct your daily duties through your mind, action and speech. EGO IS NOTHING MORE THAN THAT.

CHITTA is the storehouse of all your samskaras or impressions. When you look closer, you will understand chitta is not actually the mind but is a vast storehouse of the merits and demerits of your life. You have stored millions of impressions in the many levels of the unconscious. If you want to know what you are going to do in the future, you can know it by studying the impressions lying in the unconscious, the storehouse you have created. When you meditate, those impressions will come from the unconscious and you will have to deal with them.

Chitta is like the bottom of a lake where all the pebbles you have thrown have settled down. This can be observed externally in the early days of practice because your facial expression changes many times in response to the passing thought forms. Sometimes you smile, sometimes you become very serious and sometimes very drowsy and sleepy; and all the while you are convinced you are meditating. Once I had a cameraman take a video of some students while they were meditating. After five minutes the students were making many faces while they were supposed to be meditating because they were affected by the impressions coming up. There is a very close relationship between emotion and thought. The face is the index that tells on you. It is the index of your heart.

When a thought or image affects your heart, it will be reflected on your face.

INNER DIALOGUE

Now, you are going beyond after analyzing and understanding all the different functions of your mind. You can understand yourself by having a dialogue with yourself. You all talk to yourselves, but not honestly, sincerely or scientifically. When you understand all four functions separately and enter into a free dialogue with yourself, sometimes that dialogue will help you to go beyond. Condensed self-dialogue is prayer. *Is it my mind that is dictating the terms that are confusing me? If manas is confusing me, why should I not take help from my buddhi?* When you start to talk to yourself, you will receive all the answers, no matter how many questions you pose.

Ramdasa, one of the most important sages of India, used to begin his practice by having a dialogue with his mind before meditation: *Oh mind, please flow on the path of devotion and the path of love.* If you begin talking to your mind, then your mind will not trouble you with any image, idea or fantasy when you sit in meditation. But if you immediately sit down to meditate, then your mind will give you back the same thoughts that you have fed to your mind. You feed your mind with objects and ideas, so when you want your mind to give you back something it cannot give you anything beyond that. This is the law of karma, and you are reaping the fruits of your karma.

CONSCIOUS AND UNCONSCIOUS

Now, you will have to work with that part of mind that functions during the waking state, the conscious or objective mind. You cultivate only this small part of the totality of mind that is in the waking state, while the vast part of mind is not under your control. You cannot meditate while dreaming, during deep sleep or in the state of turiya; you can meditate only during the waking state. You have to be patient when dealing with the conscious mind and try to understand its limitations. Therefore, the conscious mind needs to be cultured and guided.

When you try to analyze your conscious mind, it appears that the unconscious is another level of the conscious mind. If this is true, why are you not aware of it? You are not aware of even the conscious mind because you do not study and train it. *Unconscious* means "no control," *conscious* means "having control." When you are doing things unconsciously, it means the unconscious habits of your mind have control over you. And when you are doing something consciously, it means conscious control is there on the motion of your lungs, mind and activities. It takes a long time to understand that the unconscious mind has control over your life. Nothing happens in the external world without first happening in the internal world. Anything that you do, you have mentally done it long before you actually do it.

Sometimes the unconscious mind simultaneously functions while you are using your conscious mind, but you are not aware of that. Suppose I have a good friend. Someone comes and speaks against my friend. My conscious mind does not accept what they are saying, because I know my friend. However, when they have gone, my unconscious mind has accepted what they were saying and tells me maybe it's true. Then the question comes, *If my friend might have done like this, why did he not tell me? I must not really know the nature of my friend.*

Now I feel very sad. It is possible that when you disagree consciously, you can accept the suggestions of someone unconsciously.

MIND CONTROL

Mind control means "to know the method of using the forces of mind." The conscious mind is only a small part of the mind. If you know the whole mind, the totality of the mind, then the part that you use in your daily life will easily come under your control. It is not good to analyze the mind too much without knowing how to train it. Mind comes in the way and creates many problems for you, but you should also remember that mind is yours; you do not belong to your mind. You can control your mind provided you understand it. To control the mind does not mean to stop the thought process. Many of you expect that mind should not function and thoughts should not come during meditation. Some students stop doing meditation when they realize they cannot control the mind during meditation. MIND WILL CONTINUE TO FUNCTION UNTIL YOU DIE. The human mind is a catalogue of thoughts, so thoughts have to come because that is the function of mind. You are a thinking being and it is your nature to think.

Even if you acquire mind control and self-control, they can make you more powerful but they cannot make you wise. That will come only when you understand the reason you are trying to control your mind. Mind control does not make you inert or desireless. Rather, it makes you creative, well balanced and skillful. Be patient with yourself in understanding your internal states and in dealing with your mind. Whereas mind can be a very good instrument if it is controlled, an uncontrolled mind can create great obstacles. A controlled mind is always in your hands and can help you to attain the happiness that comes from peace of mind.

You will understand what calmness is when you understand the relationship between the conscious and unconscious mind, the most difficult relationship in this universe to understand. Be aware that while your body and senses are your instruments; your conscious mind and unconscious mind can become your finest instruments to lead you to happiness.

If you have even a small amount of mind control, the pains that arise from the physical body can be controlled. You might have a physical disease but if you know your mind and acquire that energy within, that disease will not affect you. However, you may have a very strong body but you cannot remove even a very small amount of mental pain without understanding what mind is. It is better for you to control your mind and its modifications so you can control your body. A healthy mind is one that is not subject to disturbance, whether from the unconscious or the external world. When the conscious mind becomes ruled by undesirable emotions, fancies and fantasies, and other problems, then you lose control of the conscious mind and you cannot know the method of how to use the vast reservoir of the unconscious mind.

The vast part of mind remains unknown to you. That part of mind that dreams and sleeps is not under your control, and even that part of mind you are using now is not under your control. THE CONSCIOUS MIND IS THE GATEWAY TO THE CITY OF LIFE AND THE UNCONSCIOUS. With the help of meditation, the unconscious can become conscious. Anyone who understands all the different levels can finally expand the sea of the conscious mind. Then, there will be no difference between the conscious mind and the unconscious mind. Anyone who has trained a little bit of the conscious mind may be very well off in the world, but ONE WHO HAS TRAINED THE UNCONSCIOUS MIND IS A SAGE.

TRAIN OF THOUGHTS

After breath awareness comes a stumbling block— how to calm down the conscious mind. It is a common complaint from students that they cannot calm down the mind so they cannot meditate. Many students even complain they were calmer before they did meditation and that now the mind is creating more problems for them. This is a good sign. Before starting to do meditation, they were escaping and were not aware of the reality. Some days they say their meditation was very bad and other days it was wonderful. They say many images and symbols are coming. One image can create many faces and wear many garbs. An image can make you cry or laugh; it can tell you what is right and wrong and can control your life. And it started as a simple latent impression. When you recognize it is a simple impression that is controlling your life, you can understand how consciousness is involved with matter or how purusha is involved with prakriti. It's the same as you are involved with your images, the way your life is controlled by your imagination. Those images or impressions become symbols for you. They will come and go, but just remember you cannot stop them and you cannot stop thoughts from coming. To stop thoughts from coming is not the purpose of meditation.

BE STILL AND KNOW

You have to be patient when you are dealing with the conscious mind. Once or twice a day you should try to calm down your conscious mind. That is the first step toward meditation. Calmness is different from stillness. During calmness you can think, judge and decide. But when you are still, you cannot do anything. Only when your mind is perfectly calm and tranquil can you study things properly and see things clearly as they are.

The whole technique of meditation is based on stillness. Let the body become still, make the breath serene and the mind calm. Then allow that wisdom that can lead you to perfection to flow. In all journeys you have to move, but meditation is a journey in which you don't move yet you go ahead. The principle requirement is stillness. I am not telling you to start on this journey by immediately meditating, contemplating or praying. I am just telling you to be still. Even if you do not go beyond sitting still, it will be beneficial to you. If you persist, those initial unwanted movements of the body will settle down, and the physical stillness you experience will give you great joy. Even without meditation, a few moments of stillness will help give conscious rest to your body. Physical stillness can make you aware of the finer forces within you on many levels.

You may not want to sit quietly because you are not confident you will have peace. You are sitting because someone has told you to, but you don't know how to actually still yourself. You have heard that by sitting still you will experience joy. You don't have any personal experience of this, but you are trying on the basis of suggestions. The stillness required for meditation is different from the stillness of deep sleep where your mind withdraws itself from body consciousness and external consciousness. If you don't sleep for many days your mind will become disturbed. Though you are not aware of it, you do not know God when you are in deep sleep, even though you are very close to it. This is unconscious stillness. You need to learn how to consciously be still. Sleep is restful and relieves you from the stresses and strains of daily life. That little stillness gives you great joy. But you don't have to go to bed and put yourself in an unconscious state to take rest. Moreover, sleep gives you rest alone; it does not make you wise nor does it satisfy your intellectual curiosity or answer questions about life. When a fool goes to sleep, they come out a fool; nothing changes. Their personality is not transformed. But if you learn to sit still and regularly practise, eventually you can go to the very center from where consciousness flows. In this way you can transform your whole personality.

The stillness of meditation will give you great joy and help to relieve the tensions and stresses of daily life. The Bible says, BE STILL AND KNOW THAT I AM GOD. This means you can only know God when you learn to be still. If you sit comfortably, steadily and still, the godly part within will be revealed to you. Many of you complain that you are not getting results when you do meditation. You are not successful because you have many desires and you expect to have visions and many odd things in meditation. This means you have wants and you don't really want to meditate. If you sit with many desires in your mind, that is not called sitting for meditation. Meditation means just to be still and LET GOD REVEAL ITSELF TO YOU. When you learn to still your body and observe that stillness, an indescribable joy will come from within.

During the time of meditation, you have to keep your mind pleasantly busy or otherwise mind will keep bringing thoughts. To begin with, let mind survey the whole body from head to foot, and from the feet back up to the head. If you do this two or three times for a few days, unwanted body gestures such as twitchings and jerks will be arrested. Foolish teachers say such gestures are part of the kundalini experience. This is not true. They are simply expressions from your subtle body that resents the discipline you are imposing on it. You will observe at first that the body moves because you have never disciplined it. When this happens, you mistakenly think your kundalini is awakening, but actually you have not yet accomplished anything. You have not made any effort and yet you expect the kundalini to rise. The fact is, the body has never been disciplined, so it rebels. When you want the body to be still it moves, and those movements have nothing to do with the kundalini.

The yogis who studied the internal and external worlds understood the nature of mind. Fundamentally, the senses dissipate the mind. Mind does not want to go to the internal world because it is in the habit of running to the external world. Mind does not want to go to the world of abstract knowledge. Mind wants to continue to depend on the objects of the world because it is very sure that with the help of the senses it can relish and enjoy all situations in the external world. Though some of them may be painful, some are not. Some of them may be joyous, and some are not. But mind is not very certain it will have extraordinary experiences within. It's very difficult for a student to prepare their mind to start doing research in the interior world and to convince your mind to do meditation.

The first day you sit down to meditate you may find your mind is running here and there and you laugh about the dissipated condition of the mind. In one day you cannot expand the whole mind because you have not practised. Just stop and try again, but don't fight with your mind. Meditation should not be a battlefield. Fighting with the mind is never considered to be control, but it's important to lead mind along a certain route. You try again on the second day and you may find that mind has calmed down somewhat, but there is a limit. Because you have not practised or taught your mind to think in a particular way, initially mind may refuse to do what you want it to do. It will take time, because mind always runs toward the grooves of old habits. You become negative because you do not know how to confront the deep-rooted habits that play a great role in your life. You should not be bothered that your mind is roaming. Even if it goes somewhere, it will always come back to you. Let it go. When I asked my master how to deal with the mind he said, "If mind tells you to go there, don't go. Tell mind, 'Oh mind, if you want to go, you're free to go. But I am not going.'" If you discipline your mind, you will not have to struggle or fight for meditation. You sit for two hours and become more and more tense because you keep thinking you are not doing meditation and your mind is distracted and dissipated. You should not try to meditate if you are tired. Instead, try again at your capacity when you are relaxed.

Mind is in the habit of going to the past. Mantra says no, come back and don't fight. If you are feeling very anxious when you sit for meditation, you may want to relax, but suddenly you may be confronted with a rush of thought forms from the unconscious, the bed of memories. Unknowingly, you are allowing the unconscious mind to become active. While you are sitting in meditation those thought forms will keep coming from the unconscious bed of memory to the conscious mind. As long as you are trying to relax your conscious mind, the unconscious mind will throw out all that is kept there. And when the unconscious mind becomes active, the millions of impressions and emotions stored there start to come forward to the conscious mind, and then again you become restless. You have to know how to deal with those thought patterns. A thought comes and then another thought and then another and another. The whole day thought waves come in the ocean of the mind. This whole world is a projection of your ideas. Idea means "thought." Your thoughts are motivating you to move or make many gestures. Human creation, anything you see outside, is a projection of your thoughts. EVERY ACTION IS AN EXPRESSION OF A THOUGHT.

When you understand unlearning, you can choose what thoughts to retain and what to reject. That is control. When you study yourself, you come to know that your internal states are quite different than what you perceive yourself to be in the external world. Mind has a tendency to either become extroverted or to remain introverted. The thought forms that govern your life and modifications of your mind during that time make you introverted and you can no longer help yourself. This often happens and it doesn't help you to understand your internal states. However, when you become introverted you are not doing meditation. Meditation makes the mind inward and helps you to consciously control your mind and allow it to expand.

One of the purposes of meditation is to calm down the conscious mind, which is over-crowded by the rush coming from the unconscious level and from the outside. You say you want to do meditation but you cannot do it. You have to learn meditation slowly and gradually. With regular practice the breathing comes under control and as the practice progresses the mind becomes calm and steady. When you want to be calm and quiet, you withdraw from everyone. You no longer talk but you continue to think and to talk to the images that you have in your mind. Thought also requires a language. But the moment you are able to calm down the conscious mind, another problem comes. You may be preventing new sensations from disturbing the seemingly calm lake of the mind, but this is not yet control of the senses. Beneath there are waves that are not evident externally, but yet they are very disturbing. The following simile will help you understand. If you stand on the side of a calm lake and throw a few pebbles one by one, those pebbles will create a big bubble. Then, as they slowly settle down to the bottom of the lake, that bubble vanishes. A new thought form is like a pebble. When it goes down to the bed of memory it also creates a bubble. Once it settles down again it creates another bubble there and that bubble starts to increase and increase. You are throwing pebbles one after another into the lake of the mind and all the pebbles are settling down as impressions. Those impressions become stronger if they are repeated.

All the thought patterns you have stored remain in seed form in the bed of your memories. Only the impressions of those worries that you are interested in remain in a latent state in the bed of memories. When you calm down your conscious mind, they come forward from the unconscious. You have made your body still, your breath calm and you have withdrawn your senses, but the conscious mind has no power to deal with the roaring rush of impressions from the unconscious mind.

That is a serious problem before a meditator. This is why many people have problems with meditation. No one teaches you how to deal with those thoughts patterns. The most important part of meditation comes when you know how to deal with the rush coming forward from the unconscious to the conscious mind.

To deal with the conscious mind and its various thoughts you have to develop new unconscious activity by remembering your mantra so you are always aware of the reality within. In this way, the conscious functioning of mind will not affect you. Your mind has the habit of going to the external world with the help of the senses. If instead you keep the mind busy doing japa, it will become one-pointed and inward. But if you limit your practice to just doing japa, repeating the same thing over and over, you'll go crazy. To expand your consciousness you have to meditate. If you make sincere effort, after some time you will find the disturbances that you had to face in the beginning are no longer there — the body has become still, the breath is serene and the mind has become calm. Let your unconscious mind remain in a state of tranquillity by having awareness of the highest One. No matter where you are or what you are doing, you should be here yet there. Slowly you can progress until you finally reach the highest state where you are here and there both.

You have to maintain consciousness when you study your conscious mind and when the unconscious mind becomes active. Then, you will easily be able to purify the unconscious mind. When you understand the limitations of the conscious mind, you can try to calm it down to allow the unconscious mind to become active so those impressions hidden there can come straightforward to the conscious mind. There should be no effort to drive out whatever thoughts arise in the mind. If you reject everything, nothing will happen to you. You will not grow if you limit the act of witnessing to just watching the thought patterns. Simply let them have their play and merely recognize them with detachment, and before long you will understand them in their true character and form.

You have to have control over mind and its modifications. From the beginning, to deal with your conscious mind you should firmly determine that anything that comes in your mind during meditation should not disturb you. This way, gradually you can expand your sankalpa shakti (determination), and your conscious mind will also expand. You should let go of any image that comes so it does not affect you. The instant you give attention to those images, they will be there and they will stay for a long time. Your circumstances and your environment give you unconscious pressure and that is reflecting in your conscious mind when you are trying to meditate. You should first have the attitude that no matter what happens in life, when you sit in meditation you will sit in meditation. As long as you have conflict in your mind, it will not be possible for your mind to spontaneously flow inward. When there is no conflict in the mind, MIND SPONTANEOUSLY FLOWS INWARD ONE-POINTEDLY AND UNINTERRUPTEDLY. THAT IS MEDITATION.

OBSTACLES TO MEDITATION

You can easily find out the obstacles in the path of your enlightenment by observing your mind. You are bound to become aware of obstacles in the beginning. When you start to tread the path of the inner world, your awareness expands and the obstacles you will have to face come before you to your mental field. For example, you may become aware of how dull and lazy you are. Or you may become aware of the diseases you suffer from and the mental anguish. You may also become aware of your *samsaya*, the doubtful nature of your mind and your preoccupation with many other problems. Before that you had not understood much about your internal states or the obstacles within. If you are not aware of the obstacles, you cannot remove them. And if you do not remove them, you cannot attain the state of freedom. Patanjali doesn't talk of obstacles first. He talks about obstacles only when you have started to remember your mantra and you have started to meditate on the meaning of the sound.

You should try to control the thinking process by not allowing your thinking to go toward negativity but instead guiding it toward positivity. Even though you don't want to remember, worry or be involved with what is coming from the unconscious, more and more thoughts come. This is natural. Just have patience and allow all those thought forms to come to your conscious mind without fighting with your mind. You come to know very late that there is something that suddenly upsets your emotional life and then completely controls your life. If it is positive, you say it is an angel and if it is negative, you call it the devil. When you start to study the angel and devil parts of your unconscious mind, one day you realize both are within you. You can shun the part that is negative and encourage the positive part.

SENSATIONS

Unless you change the conscious mind, it will not be possible for you to study the unconscious mind. You might talk on the basis of Freudian philosophy or give quotations from Jung, Adler, James and other psychologists, but this doesn't mean you understand how the objective mind functions. When you see, hear, smell, taste or touch something, it affects you. The conscious mind always gives importance to the sensations you receive according to your interest. Then, it finally filters those sensations as impressions that go to your unconscious mind. Any sensations that you receive have to go through the filter of the conscious mind. Only the impressions of those worries that you are interested in remain in a latent state in the bed of memories. When the interest increases, because of repeated actions and thoughts, they become stronger, though they are in the form of impressions. A small impression that you keep in your unconscious mind such as hatred for someone can grow to become so strong till one day you may even try to kill that person.

Now, I want to discuss feelings, emotions and thinking. Where does the mind come from and how do feelings come? What is the difference between feelings and thoughts? You all think and understand, but that understanding is not more powerful than feelings and emotions. You cannot have any emotions without feelings. And if you do not feel anything, you cannot think at all. Feeling in a way is a blind thing and that is why it is compared with a blind man who can walk but who doesn't know the right direction to walk. When you make sense contact with the objects of the world they give you sensations, and when you receive sensations you feel something. But feelings in their primitive state are very dangerous unless they consult the mind and go through the process of filtration. The coffee granules you put in the coffee percolator will demonstrate how your mind functions. You don't drink the coffee that you put in the percolator. It has to first go through a process of filtration and then you drink the coffee that is percolated down below. Similarly, the CONSCIOUS MIND ACTS AS A FILTER. You receive sensations all the time through the five cognitive senses, and these sensations are filters. Life is a burden because you do not know how to handle the sensations you are receiving all the time. It can be stopped if you understand how you are receiving the sensations. When the senses contact matter, you can receive one of three types of sensations: pleasure, pain or neither painful or pleasant. For example, when you go from your home to your office, you may see many trees. You cannot see a tree if you have no sensation of seeing. But that doesn't give you either pain or pleasure. But if you see a friend and you smile, that pleases you. Or if you see somebody who annoys you every day, that gives you pain. So contact of the senses with the objects of the world brings sensations that are pleasurable, painful or neither pleasurable nor painful. Anytime that I look at you, my optic nerve receives your form, takes it to my brain, then to my conscious mind and finally to my unconscious mind where it is stored as an image. Now, if I don't see you for some time and then I see you again, I recognize you because I have stored your image in my unconscious. That reminds me that I have seen you before. So that reservoir within you, where you store the merits and demerits of your life, is vast. You are trying to understand that part of mind, but for the time being it is better to just deal with your conscious mind.

These sensations are being carried and then supplied to different parts of the body as needed. If you know how to disconnect from sense contact you will not have fresh sensations. But those sensations you have already stored in the basement of your unconscious mind remain there, waiting for the opportunity to be expressed. And when the opportunity comes, they become active and go to their proper places. If that sensation is connected to food, it will go to the food fountain and will remain there. If it is concerning sleep, it will be there. If it is concerning fear, it will be there. If it is concerning sex, it will be there. And when the opportunity comes, those emotions arise.

When you have stored a sensation in your unconscious mind, that sensation might create an impression that is similar to a former impression, and thus will create the same sensation or a feeling of similar quality. And the bubble that comes up from the bottom of the lake of the mind will also have similar qualities. When it comes up it will grow until it finally bursts onto the surface of the lake of mind, and then you will find similar effects of the same bubble.

Lately, medical science has come to understand the importance of relaxation. However, they are still focused on releasing muscle tension because they don't understand that the real source of stress and strain in human life is the unconscious mind. When you learn to relax the conscious mind, the unconscious immediately becomes active. And there are many levels of the unconscious mind. For knowing the various levels of life, you will have to grow and understand all the levels of your being. And for that you will have to train and lead your mind. It is best to withdraw the mind whenever it wanders away due to the attraction of various objects of the senses or memory.

You can accidentally come in touch with the various faculties within you but you should not be swayed by that. You will have to systematically avoid all these disturbances and not be satisfied with all these experiences. Suddenly you may find consciousness fading, and you might go toward a daydreaming state, or forgetfulness. Ordinarily, when the conscious mind is not working and the unconscious remains conscious, consciousness fades, because it has no power to remain all alone without the use of the conscious mind. Then, it starts to dream. The dreams come because you have stored many previous experiences and impressions of the objective world within the reservoir of the unconscious. In meditation, you can consciously cut off from the conscious mind but still maintain consciousness and allow those impressions to come forward and to consciously let them go. This is the way you can exhaust the entire fund of impressions that are lying dormant in the unconscious. But when you practise, you will find that you can easily watch all the impressions you have stored in the unconscious mind by maintaining consciousness. When this happens, you will find that you are touching a point that is beyond your transpersonal mind.

LETTING GO

When you start to work with your unconscious mind, a time comes when you think you might lose your mind. Suddenly one day, for no rhyme or reason, you think, *I might die! What will happen if I die tomorrow? What will happen if I get sick and nobody is there to look after me?* You come in touch with negative fears such as these that remain hidden in the unconscious. One day you are smiling for no reason; the next day you are feeling very sad because of the interference of those impressions that are hidden in the memory. Patanjali said these should also be controlled, and with the help of meditation, you can do it. Images come and it is difficult for you to let go of those images. You should talk to those images: *How are you coming into my mind? This is the time for meditation. When the right time comes, I will recall you. Please see me when I am not meditating. Problems and images should not come to me when I am meditating.* You need to form the habit of letting thoughts come and go away. Have the determination that you will let go of any image that comes. It doesn't mean you are to be indifferent; you are just allowing them to go away.

First, you have to become aware of the thoughts. Then, determine that you will not brood on any thought that comes into your mind. As soon as you close your eyes, you should have the attitude that no matter what comes in your mind, you will just allow it to go. Let go of whatever image or thought that comes in your mind without allowing them to affect you. Whatever thoughts or concepts or obscuring passions arise in the mind they are not to be driven out or allowed to control you; simply let them have their play without any effort to direct them. When they arise, merely recognize them with detachment and before long you will understand them in their true character and form.

Let go of the thought patterns coming from the unconscious, because they are not yours; they have come from outside. Only that which you have seen, heard, thought of, studied, imagined or dreamt of can come in your mind during meditation. Don't allow thought patterns to upset you or your mind. Meditation will help you to learn how to not identify with those thought patterns. Just allow all the thoughts to continue without identifying with them. When you identify with your thought patterns you forget your true Self. For the first few days you may find problems, just like any other new thing you undertake. But if you regularly practise for some time, you will be able to do it.

You have to attend to your ceaseless involvement with your mental activity, emotions and thoughts. When you think of something, you take action and you assume that you are 100 percent right. Your reason is not always in control of all your actions. Usually, you just do them. This will not happen if do not identify yourself with the objects of your mind. Your thoughts lead you—your mind, action and speech—the way they want so they can control you. This is why you have to watch your thinking process. You can decide that whatever comes into your mind, you will just let it go. In order to do that, you will need a point of focus for the mind. Suddenly something comes in your mind because of past experiences and samskaras, and again the mind will bring you back. Just keep remembering your mantra and reminding yourself that any thought that comes is insignificant. If your mind repeatedly remembers the mantra, it will create a deep groove in the mind. The difference between an ordinary person and a sage is this: An ordinary person with an untrained mind does not know how to let go; they are affected by their thoughts and by someone else's actions and words. But a sage who has trained their mind knows how to let go of thoughts so mind is not affected by them at all.

Very few people know how to study thought patterns, because it is personal experience, and there are no books on the subject. However, thought patterns can be studied through biofeedback. If you are thinking in a certain way, it will create a particular pattern on the screen of the machine. It's a very interesting study to find out why you are creating particular patterns. You have to nourish those thought patterns or feelings that are helpful, and reject those that are not helpful. Accepting and rejecting — that is life. You reject that which is not needed all the time.

When you do that, your mind becomes one-pointed and inward. That is dharana.

WITNESSING

Next is to observe the thinking process without getting involved. When you begin to meditate the first thing you find out is that you cannot meditate, because mind remains preoccupied. Even if you do all the necessary preliminaries, when mind is preoccupied it is difficult to meditate. As you try to calm down your conscious mind, the unconscious mind automatically becomes very active and many vrittis come up from the basement. For that there is only one method to deal with all the samskaras that come forward: YOU HAVE TO BE THE SEER AND LEARN TO WITNESS.

It is very important to understand what happens when you witness things: *I am not the body, I am not the breath, I am not the senses, I am not the mind.* Now you are witnessing and you have become a seer. You see things separately from yourself. This is one of the steps of meditation. When you learn to witness, you will begin to see things properly. But if you are involved in something, you cannot witness it because you assume the form and identify yourself with the object. For witnessing you will have to learn this process, *I am not this, I am not this, I am not this.* This is called *neti neti,* NOT THIS, NOT THIS.

Allow your thoughts to come forward from the unconscious and witness them instead of brooding on them. If your mind does not brood on the thoughts you will remain unaffected as you let go of your thoughts. You should develop an attitude of complete detachment toward your actions and thoughts so you can have absolute peace of mind. Attainment of a detached state of being in which one is only an observer and not a doer will lead to complete relaxation of mind and body. Then you can learn to focus the mind one-pointedly.

The next step is to observe the train of thoughts. One should not fight the train of thoughts that is incessantly rising in the mind or try to suppress them, but should quietly observe them. It is a little difficult to do so in the beginning, but it becomes easier with constant practice. It's interesting to watch that part of mind you are trying to train and educate and that part of mind that is helping you to do this. You will find the conscious part of mind is slowly expanding. You allow all the thoughts to come forward from the unconscious mind and you simply observe them and don't get involved. If anything comes into your mind, and if you do not accept it within the mind, then it is not yours. Even the realization that a thought does not belong to you involves the thought of someone else. What is that thought that is your thought? No thought is really yours. In all of your thoughts, there is someone else involved, or there is an image from outside. Gradually you will catch hold of that part of mind that is not normally under your control.

You should not allow thought patterns to disturb you. They will come before one who does meditation and one who does not do meditation. Simply witness your thinking process. This is a key point. When you truly witness something then you can really enjoy and understand it. But when you get involved and you identify yourself with the thoughts, then you forget your true Self. Be patient with yourself and persist in your efforts so you gradually expand your capacity. Never give up or say you cannot train yourself. With the help of training, you can change the grooves of your mind and help yourself. Be vigilant. In this way you will find that the myriad of thoughts that are coming from the unconscious where you have stored many impressions from your daily life will not affect you. You are simply being a witness. During that time your mind, nervous system, muscles and all the tissues and cells will get perfect rest. Even if you cannot go beyond that, it's very healthy to sit still.

The same process goes on in the first stage of meditation. When thought patterns come and go through the mental train, you will find that some of the thought patterns are helpful and some are not because they create disturbance. The important thing is not to get involved with them. Don't allow the unconscious mind to disturb the conscious mind. You should allow the mind to go on with its thinking process, but don't let it disturb you. Even though you do not want to remember, or worry or think, more things will come from the unconscious during those times. If you understand this, then you will understand you have to have the patience to allow all those thought forms to come to your conscious mind and just let them go. Then, they will never come back. Let each thought come, whether it is good or bad. Just decide that whatever comes, you will not be disturbed. Realize that this thought, whatever it is, cannot disturb your whole life. To think otherwise means you think you are weak and thought is very powerful. What happens to most people is that any thought that comes into their mind disturbs their whole being. Then another thought comes, and that also disturbs them, and this happens continuously. Then they become weak and spineless when such thoughts come. They remain afraid because more thoughts are coming into their mind. Suddenly they realize this, get upset and ask themselves why they are thinking like this.

The difference between you and an accomplished swami is this: you take things into your heart, but a swami doesn't. You could tell a swami, "Hey, Swami, you are a fool," and they would never take it to heart. They don't take in such suggestions so easily. On the other hand, you take in everything. If a swami were to tell you that you were a fool, then you might leave and never come back. You are easily influenced by others' suggestions because you have not yet built your personality. The day that you build your own personality, you will no longer be moved by another person's suggestions.

To establish strength, decide that whatever thought occurs, or whatever others say, you will not accept it blindly. You will just observe it and let it come. One person may tell you that you are going to die tomorrow. Perhaps another person tells you that you will become a powerful person. These two thoughts may come together. One thought is flattering to your ego, but the other thought is crippling your will power. Allow both kinds of thoughts to come. Be conscious of them. Remember that whatever thought comes, a thought is only a thought. Why should you allow that thought to affect you? It will affect you only when you accept it. You can observe such thoughts without accepting them as your own.

Before I practice meditation, I allow all such thoughts, both good and bad, to come into my mind and then go away, because they are only thoughts. Try to think of any thought that you can keep in your mind forever. It is not possible. A thought is that which comes into the mind and goes away. Why should a thought that merely comes and goes away lead or influence your life? Most of the time, if it is a bad thought you feel bad. Instead, you should just allow it to leave. You can control both the bad and good thoughts that leave imprints in your mind; let them merely come and then go away. If these thoughts are not fulfilled, they lose power and die. This is the practice of self-psychiatry.

Perhaps a thought comes into my mind and tells me, *Come on, steal this glass.* My mind can say, *My dear thought, if you want to steal it, go ahead, but I am not going with you.* Then what happens? The thought will pass without my stealing anything. The first step is to let that thought come and pass. Even if you want to keep a thought in your mind, you cannot. Another thought comes and will push it aside. If you think of your husband, then next you will suddenly think of your child. Then you will think of your house and your car. So many thoughts come and go. Each thought is pushed by another in a continuous train of thoughts. Just let them go away.

If one particular thought comes and goes again and again, and if you do not take any action, then what happens to it? It will eventually not continue to come back, because you are not paying it any interest. Those thoughts that are colored by your interest and attention are the ones that motivate you to do things. Not all thoughts have that power. Not all of your thoughts need expression externally, so allow your thoughts to arise, decide if they are creative or helpful thoughts and then express those that are useful.

The first lesson in this practice is to simply allow the thoughts to arise. Then, bring back that which is important. You can easily do this; it does not require any advanced practice of yoga. Usually, however, something important will come to you and either you start to worry or you start to enjoy your imagination. Do not form the habit of enjoying your thinking process and indulging in it without action; such daydreaming is very dangerous. That is not the same as creative imagination. Creative imagination is that process by which you imagine something and then allow it to be expressed through your actions when it is helpful.

When all the thoughts have passed through the mind, then start to remember your mantra. Even though there are some thoughts waiting for your consultation, do not pay attention to them. The thoughts are coming and going in your mind, while you are repeating your mantra. The more they come, the more you repeat your mantra, and then there seems to be an internal battle taking place. That is not helpful; you should not do that.

Mind creates the space; meditation will fill up all that space so there will be uninterrupted awareness. Beneath all those thoughts you have to maintain awareness of the center of reality within. When you reach the deeper states of meditation, you will still think, but the difference is you will not be affected by those thoughts. When you have learned to witness for a long time the thought forms coming from the unconscious without being affected by them, then the thought forms will come and go, and there will not be a single expression on your face or gesture of your body. To reach this point, first, you will have to learn to not allow the external world and sensations to stimulate or disturb you. Next, you cannot allow yourself to be affected by the impressions stored in the unconscious. And finally, you can go beyond and maintain a state of tranquillity.

INTROSPECTION

Once you have learned not to identify with the thought patterns then you have to start the process of introspection, or inspecting within. In this state, you are not being influenced by the thought patterns and you are not identifying with them; you are remaining detached. The faculty of introspection should be sharpened so much so that you understand which thought pattern should be allowed and which should not be allowed. That is an advanced stage of witnessing. In simple witnessing you don't inspect. You inspect only when you have the power to inspect all the symbols running through the train of thoughts. Once you have that power you determine you will not get involved with those samskaras, no matter what happens. The first time you try, you may perhaps have two per cent success; the second time, perhaps five per cent. Slowly you will learn to isolate yourself from your thoughts so you no longer identify with them. Then you will be in charge of yourself and will no longer be randomly led by your thought patterns.

TYPES OF THOUGHT PATTERNS

There are three types of thought patterns: helpful, disturbing and another that is neither helpful nor obstacle. This is the way to start the practice of introspection, or inspecting. First, you should learn to not allow any external stimuli, sensations, sounds or anything else to disturb you when you sit down in meditation. Second, you should allow all thought forms to go away. Third, you should learn which particular thought form is helpful for you and which is not. And fourth, you should learn to strengthen those thought forms that are helpful and discourage those that are not helpful.

You can understand the value of thought patterns by examining them: *Why is this particular thought pattern coming to me again and again? Which part of me is related to that? Why do I hate that person? Which part of me is related to this hatred? How do they disturb me? If I hate someone, it means I am definitely weak. I should accept that I am weak. I hate them because they have a different religion. Though I understand my religion, I do not understand theirs and I don't want to understand it.* This is all due to an ego problem. Another is a cultural problem. If I dress in a particular style, and you don't like that style, my reaction is to not like your dress. So, we cannot communicate. Third is the problem of interest. I have a particular value for a thing. I like this thing this way, but you want it to be a different way. Or you don't want to share my hobby and I don't want to share yours. Don't strengthen your weakness more and more by expanding your hatred. It can bring on mental problems and can create a psychosomatic problem. It can become a source of constant trouble within you. Just understand that any particular thought form is a source of distraction to your mind. You should study what it is, why it is a source of distraction to your mind and how it is related to a particular emotional problem. That is why it keeps coming to you again and again. Sometimes the object of love is less powerful than the object of hatred. If you hate somebody you remember them more and more. That is also concentration. And you do it so much, even if you do not want to. You become helpless when you hate somebody.

One who meditates becomes more aware of their thought patterns and knows from which level those thought patterns are arising. Are they worldly? Are they without guidance or are they well managed thoughts? Are they only imaginations or hallucinations? Don't waste your time in hallucinations or in analyzing thought patterns. Meditation time is not meant for thinking or worrying; it's meant for meditation. It is better not to analyze them during meditation time or else your whole time will be consumed. It is better to focus your mind on only one thought pattern instead of allowing your mind to run here and there. Meditation is a system that helps you to study yourself. It is not hallucination, imagination or sitting and worrying, nor is it a means of pampering yourself and feeding your fantasies. Mind can imagine, but imagination is not meditation. If you are imagining an image and you are brooding on an image you have seen in the past, that is not meditation.

To become thoughtless is not possible. During meditation, you don't have thoughtlessness; you should have only one thought in your mind. And all other thoughts should be swallowed by that particular thought, exactly like a wave of the ocean swallows all smaller waves because it is stronger. When all the little thoughts coming and going unite to make one deep, powerful wave, mind flows with one-pointedness and such a powerful one-pointed mind is capable of fathoming the deeper levels of your being and can lead you to the other shore of life from where it has come. The mind that has become inward and one-pointed is very helpful and can lead you beyond the gross world so you can tread the path of light. For that, your whole being will become an eye and then you will truly see, but not with the two eyes. You will remain in a state of sleepless sleep and tranquillity; you will become a *drishta*, where you can see everything. But it is never said that the mind can show you God.

Many times a sadhaka on the path of enlightenment may think they have known everything there is to know and therefore they are free. But a bubble may suddenly arise from the lake of the mind because somebody annoys you and you become disturbed. You should learn to relax so that when you want to remember, it should flow directly. If you observe your thought patterns and do not become involved mentally with them, slowly you will find your mind is becoming inward toward the unconscious mind. It's a very interesting experience. In the beginning you might feel sleepy and spacey. Gradually expand the time you spend sitting. If you can meditate for ten minutes without any interruption, you will attain a state of samadhi. There is no need to hallucinate for two hours and then claim nothing is happening. Either you were sleeping, hallucinating or counting your thoughts but you were not meditating. Don't waste so much time uselessly. On the path of enlightenment, do not ever feel that you have known everything.

INNER LIGHT AND INNER SOUNDS

You should remain aware of the center of consciousness where the inner light and inner sounds are inseparable. A sadhaka has a choice according to their inherent tendencies. Either they should strengthen visualization or they should engage the mind in listening to the sounds coming from within. One of these two tendencies is predominant in every individual. For some, visualization is easy; for others, it is easier to listen. If you want to visualize when you meditate, concentrate on the breath flow and what color it is. The actual color of prana is *prakasha,* or light. Colors come because of the *tattwas* (elements). There are five tattwas: earth *(prithvi),* water *(apas),* fire *(agni),* air *(vayu)* and ether *(akasha).* Each tattwa has its color. When earth is active, you will see a dull light; if you sense a fragrance, it means you are one with the prithvi tattva at that time, because fragrance is a quality of the prithvi tattva. When you begin to practise meditation, lights may come and disappear according to the predominance of the tattvas. When one of the tattwas changes or becomes predominant, the color of the image will change. One day you may see a golden light; another day a different light. That is not indicative of progress. First, you may see a light, and suddenly you'll find it is becoming red. Then again it will change and become blue. But prana is beyond the tattwas. If you have trained your prana, it will not allow the color to change. You have to establish harmony to prevent any particular tattwa from being dominant. Otherwise, the predominance of a tattwa will not allow you to go beyond.

If you pay attention to your breath flow in a calm and still posture, you will find that your breath whispers a song and so does your brain. The heart also has a particular rhythm that is perfect music. Nada is a sound heard from within during meditation. When you can hear the sounds of the flow of prana within, then you discover there are different levels of nada. For example, initially you may become aware of the sounds from the prana flowing in your nerves. Then, you may hear different subtle sounds from the flow of prana right from the medulla to your pelvic plexus. Your mind is being led by mantra toward the silence. And finally, you reach the state from where all nadas are coming, and that is the most silent state of nada.

When an aspirant is able to make his whole being into an ear, they can hear the unstruck sounds of anahata nada that come from the silence within. Meditation helps you to hear these sounds systematically. Initially, you will hear the grosser inner sounds that are coming to your consciousness. As your mind becomes more and more concentrated, you will start to hear the finer sounds with the ear of your mind. The first sound resembles the dropping of a nail on the floor. Next, a whistling sound comes followed by a sound that resembles trumpets. Then, the very melodious sound of a flute comes along with the sound of a string instrument. In the end, many string instruments are heard all at the same time. Finally, you will hear a sound like OM and your whole being will vibrate from within though your body remains still.

When your mind is not following the subtle sound of the mantra, then it becomes aware of the illumination of ajna chakra. This prevents the mind from running toward external objects. Suddenly your mind enters into something like a tunnel that leads you to the gateway to sahasrara chakra, the thousand-petalled lotus. This particular gate according to the yogis is called the tenth gate in the city of life. No external sound or disturbance is able to distract you at this stage. On the way you may find many experiences and visions. Sometimes you will receive a hunch, sometimes thoughts may flash from the source of intuition. You might experience colorful sparks of light and strange sounds such as thundering clouds. These experiences help to create confidence in the mind of the student so they become more inclined toward the practice. If one day you experience something and the next day you don't, you should not be disappointed. This happens because the mind remains distracted and still has a tendency to flow into the past grooves of memory. After doing meditation for more than 30 minutes in one position you will be able to observe the roaming habits of your mind and its hidden tendencies. You can gradually eliminate them and cross the final boundary built by your mind within you. When depression and anxiety reduce considerably, and calmness and fearlessness increase, you can be sure that you are progressing. This gradual process of self-transformation helps to increase your awareness.

By meditating regularly at the same time every day the mind forms the habit of dwelling in the inner world and rejoices in having unusual visions. But all visions are not unalloyed. They are often mingled with fantasies, hallucinations and confusion. Intuitive knowledge is unalloyed knowledge that does not need any support or proof. At this stage many times the intellect runs to the factual world or it recalls previous experiences stored in the unconscious. It is better for the true student of meditation to discard all such experiences without being affected.

You have to judge yourself by studying the trends of your mind. You should talk to your teacher about your inner tendencies and the observations you find in your meditation. Whether it visualizes or listens to the sounds coming from within, a one-pointed and inward mind is powerful and can penetrate into the inner dimensions and unfold your interior states.

MIND POWER

When you have complete command over your mind and its modifications, you will be able to go to the unconscious easily and tap the bed of your memories. This will enable you to use the selected memory in your daily life. Then, you will have proper judgment and you will understand the importance of what you have to do, when you should do it and why you are doing it.

You put so much value on things, whereas in reality they don't have any power at all. Because you have not yet understood your internal states, you don't realize the actual power lies in your mind. Even a distracted mind could become very powerful and very destructive. Once you become aware of the power of your mind, you will have to curb that power. The meditative sciences suggest that the mind has vast powers of memory, understanding, intuition and knowledge that most persons can only glimpse. Occasionally, there may be some incidental evidence of these abilities, but when this occurs such experiences are usually explained as illusory or coincidental.

A taste for something higher comes when you do meditation. Even if you apply all the knowledge you have acquired up to this time, there is a faculty within you that wants to know more and more. Acquired knowledge does not bring satisfaction because you have not known the real issues of life. What does it mean to know something? How do you know something, and when you know it, how do you know that you know it? When you have some understanding of anything in the world, you have to take that knowledge through the process of filtration and analysis before you can declare you know it. What you call *knowing* is the sum of knowledge that has been received from various quarters within and without, after experimentation and full of experience. You should learn to depend only on inner knowledge, because your mind plays tricks with you, and then suddenly you start to lose self-confidence. The moment you lose self-confidence, your mind cannot decide anything in time. And if you miss what you have to do today and try to do it tomorrow, it will not be the same.

After some time, you will find that instead of going outward mind will start to go inward. You are trying to direct your conscious mind toward the unconscious, to the reservoir within. Naturally, you will have to face all the memories, good and bad. *Bad* is that which disturbs you, *good* is that which is helpful in life. In the beginning you will have to learn not to be swayed by good or bad, but just to let go. All mental tensions arise from the unconscious because all the information received through the conscious mind is stored in the unconscious mind. You have to decide not to allow your mind to be swayed because the Lord is within you. When you are trying to calm down the conscious mind, naturally the unconscious mind will become active. But you have to go through this to understand the whole mind. Superficial things you forget, but deep samskaras you cannot forget. A time will come when you will understand the reservoir of samskaras. Only then will you be able to go beyond that. So DON'T GIVE UP, LEARN TO BE STILL. The knowledge that comes from within will come of itself.

At this point in the practice of meditation, the body is relaxed, the conscious mind is relaxed and the impressions that are stored in the unconscious mind are coming. You have many varieties of impressions. You store those impressions that you love or hate. Sometimes hatred is stronger than love. Those impressions are already there, so they will come. If you have decided you will not allow your mind to be swayed, you can observe but not get attached to those impressions. You should decide that anything that comes in your mind during that time, you will just let it go. Go beyond and watch your thinking process. When a thought comes, let it go. This is the way you can get freedom from the impressions you have stored in the unconscious.

MEDITATION PRACTICUMS

MEDITATION PRACTICUM NO. 1

Now, I want to give you systematic instructions so you can properly meditate. If you are sitting on the floor use a folded blanket or cushion; if you prefer to sit on a chair, place your hands on your thighs, keeping your head, neck and trunk aligned. Do not over stretch your spinal column. Gently close your eyes. The body should be relaxed.

Pay attention to the flow of your breath. See that you are not creating jerks, you are not breathing shallowly, you are not pausing between the two breaths and that you are breathing according to your comfortable capacity. Remember to gently seal your lips and breathe through the nostrils only. Let your mind flow gently and smoothly with the breath.

Now, you will enjoy true relaxation that is based on the breathing system and not on hypnosis. To relax does not mean to loosen the muscles; it means "to let go of tension." Push in your upper abdomen and exhale. Push in as much as you can comfortably, watching the capacity of your lungs. Don't overdo. Gently exhale and let the air come out and then start inhaling again. When you exhale the consumed air, it will relax your nervous system. Do not suggest anything to your mind. Exhale as though you are exhaling all your problems; inhale the vital energy prana.

Exhale as though you are exhaling from the crown of your head down to the toes, relaxing as you exhale; inhale as though you are inhaling energy from the toes up to the crown of your head. Exhale as though you are exhaling all toxins and all problems, inhale as though you are inhaling vital energy. Breathe as though your whole body is exhaling and inhaling. Your mind is flowing spontaneously with the flow of the breath, and you are completely relaxed. Feel as though your whole body has become very light and is floating in the air.

Do not suggest anything to your mind; just observe the whole body systematically from head to toe. As you are quickly examining the whole body, the mind will stop where it comes across any tension. Let go of any tension from your scalp, forehead, eyes, cheeks and jaws. Release all tension from your neck, shoulders, arms, hands and fingers; then chest, abdomen, pelvis, thighs, knees, calf muscles, ankles and feet. Release all tension from your whole body.

Breathe in a serene way and observe your thinking process. Decide you are not going to identify with the thought patterns that are coming in your mind.

If you are in the habit of remembering your mantra with the inhalation and exhalation, you can inhale your mantra and without any retention exhale your mantra. Inhale and exhale your mantra. Always consult your teacher first, because there are mantras that are not coordinated with inhalation and exhalation. A mantra is a soothing sound that vibrates as it strengthens and relaxes your nervous system. These sounds were experienced in deep states of meditation by the great sages and are known by their particular vibrations.

Let your mind remember your mantra. If the mind runs here and there and goes back to the old grooves of your habits or memories, do not worry. You can bring it back. Gently remember the mantra again and let your mind follow the sound of your mantra with one-pointedness. Your mind is following the mantra and going toward the silence, gently crossing the individual boundaries of thinking and feeling. Mind has immense capacity to act the way you train it. The mantra is leading your mind toward the center of your being, the center of your consciousness, which is the fountainhead of silence.

In the path of meditation, you will fathom the different levels of consciousness, one by one, until you reach the fountainhead of pure divinity, happiness and joy (satyam shivam sundaram). The subtle feeling of your mantra remains so your mind and your mantra become one. The feeling of mantra and awareness will still be there. A good person is naturally aware of truth the whole day because they do not do anything that goes against truth. They do not have to keep repeating truth, truth, truth because they understand what truth is.

Your mind is observing and witnessing the silence within you. Deep down within you lies the center of peace, happiness and wisdom. Your mind is becoming one-pointed and inward and is enjoying the glory of the silence. When you have trained your mind, and mind has fathomed the subtlest aspects of your being and internal states, a time will come where you will become one with your essential nature that is peace, happiness and wisdom. You will be like a wave of joy in the eternal ocean of bliss. Once you have realized this you will find peace and happiness within and without and you will be free from all fears. When you come to know the center of consciousness, the center of peace, happiness, and wisdom is within you, you will be confident enough to know it is not beyond your reach. So far you have been identifying with the objects of the mind. But now you know that the objects of the mind have nothing to do with your essential nature.

Again you are remembering your mantra. Your mind is in a perfect state of tranquillity and equanimity. The more your mind follows the subtle sounds of your mantra, the more creative and dynamic it becomes. The more your mind goes toward silence, the more it soothes your nervous system and strengthens your vitality. Your mantra is radiating love, fearlessness and strength. Do not worry if your mind runs here and there. Remember your mantra and again inhale and exhale your mantra. Do not interrupt the mantra but just exhale one mantra and start inhaling without consciously creating any pause.

Now, you no longer hear the sound of your mantra. Mantra and mind are becoming one as mind is following the mantra with its full attention. Exhale as though you are exhaling from the crown of your head down through your toes and inhale as though you are inhaling the vital force from the atmosphere. You are filling up your whole being with the vital force that is given to you by the cosmic consciousness. When you exhale you are releasing all stress, strain and fatigue. Continue to remember your mantra with your breath. Form the habit of being conscious of your mantra all the time. Mantra is a compact prayer. You are inhaling the mantra and exhaling the mantra. There is no sound coming out of your nostrils, there are no jerks and no noise in your breath; your breath is deep and you are not creating a pause between inhalation and exhalation. When you have withdrawn voluntarily from the external world, focus your mind on the breath and mantra and you will experience peace. The center of peace is within you and there is peace without. Your mind is becoming one-pointed and inward. Your mind is observing and witnessing the silence within you and is enjoying the glory of the silence.

Here, you should remember that you are not only a body. You are different from the body that is your grossest instrument. You also have senses and your senses are also different from you. Your senses are your finer instruments. The body is your grossest instrument, the breath and senses are subtler and the subtlest is your mind. You are not only a body and a breathing being, but you are a thinking being too. You have a mind, you are thinking, feeling and desiring, but you are different from your body, senses and mind. These are your instruments, but who are you? You are seated behind and beyond mind, senses, breath and body. You are different from your instruments so you should not identify with them. You are a ripple of joy in the ocean of bliss. You were born out of this ocean, you play in this ocean and finally, you will merge into this ocean. You will never die because you are an immortal child of eternity. Death belongs to the physical body, breath, senses and mind only. There is no death for you for you are a child of eternity, a beloved child of the Lord. You should remember this in all walks of life, wherever you go. Try to be constantly aware of the truth within. You are a shrine of the Lord. Not only is the Lord in you, the Lord is everywhere. You are experiencing joy and happiness.

Now, very gently move your fingers. Remembering your mantra, continue to breathe smoothly and evenly. When you feel ready, gently open your eyes.

OM, shanti, shanti, shanti.
Peace, peace, peace.

MEDITATION PRACTICUM NUMBER 2

OM poorna madhaha
Poorna midam poornat poorna mudhaschyathe
Poornasya poorna madaya poorna meva vasishyathe
From Isho Upanishad

What is visible is the infinite.
What is invisible is also the infinite.
Out of the Infinite Being the finite has come,
yet being infinite, only the infinite remains.

OM shanti, shanti, shanti.
Peace, peace, peace.

Gently close your eyes, keeping your head, neck and trunk straight. Place your hands on your thighs. Ask your mind to observe the whole body from head to toe. Mind can easily know which part of the body is tense. Ask your mind to relax. Relax does not mean to loosen the muscles; *to relax* means "to release all tension." Tell your mind to systematically examine your body from head to toe. If your scalp, forehead, eyes, cheeks and jaw are relaxed, then relax your neck, shoulders, arms, hands and fingers; relax your chest and abdomen. Relax your pelvis, thighs, knees, calf muscles, ankles and feet. Release all tension from your whole body.

Now, pay attention to your breath, for breath is life and life is breath. See that your breath is deep and silent, with no jerks or pauses. Your breath should be serene and smooth. When you breathe according to your comfortable capacity, your muscles and nervous system become relaxed. Just be aware that you are breathing systematically using your diaphragm, not creating jerks but breathing freely and smoothly.

Exhale as though you are exhaling all toxins; then, inhale energy from the atmosphere. Then, exhale as though you are exhaling from the crown of your head down to the toes, relaxing the whole body. Inhale as though you are inhaling energy from the toes up to the crown of your head. Your whole body feels as if it is floating in the air. Watch your diaphragmatic movement. Push in your upper abdomen when you exhale; let it come out when you inhale. There should be no object or thought in the mind as you watch the movement of your diaphragm. Exhale and push in your diaphragm so that the diaphragm helps your lungs to expel carbon dioxide. Let it come out comfortably and inhale. You are inhaling vital energy and exhaling all wastes. Your breath is becoming smoother. Breathe as though all your pores are inhaling and exhaling.

You are not only a physical body and a breathing being, but you are also a thinking being. The body is gross, your breath and senses are subtler and mind is the subtlest. These instruments are yours, but who are you? You are seated behind and beyond mind, breath and body. You have a body and body is your instrument. You have senses; senses are your finer instruments. You have a mind, which is your finest instrument. You are not body, senses and mind, but they are your instruments. Your very existence lies beyond your mind. Your true nature is peace, happiness and wisdom.

You tend to identify with the objects of your mind. You have desires in the mind and they are colored by adjectives like good and bad. Don't identify with your mind, breath or body. You are a ripple of joy and bliss in the ocean, the almighty and absolute truth. You were born out of this ocean, you play in this ocean and eventually you will merge into this ocean. You are immortal, a child of immortality and eternity. You will never die. Death belongs to the physical body, breath and mind. There is no death for you for you are a child of eternity. Remember this in all walks of life, wherever you go.

Once in a day put yourself in a situation where you are calm, quiet, still and in deep silence. We all are children of the silence and will go back to the silence. In the beginning was the word, and the word was God, and God was the word. **THAT BEGINNING WAS SILENCE.** There you will dwell in your majesty and splendor with all joy. That is your happiness and your true nature. Breathe deeply and pay attention toward the flow of your breath. Gently open your eyes.

I pray to the divinity in you. God bless you.

MEDITATION PRACTICUM NUMBER 3

Now, I will give you a practical lesson. Sit on a cushion or a wooden chair and place your hands on the thighs. Any posture that allows you to be comfortable and steady is good. Practise the same posture everyday so that the posture does not become a source of distraction to you. Those who sit on the floor should practise an easy cross-legged posture in the beginning. Those sitting on a chair should sit with both feet apart on the floor, placing their hands on their thighs or near their knees. In all positions the head, neck and trunk should be in a straight line. Make sure your spinal cord is not crooked or stressed beyond your capacity so that you don't feel uncomfortable. How you fold the upper and lower extremities has nothing to do with posture. Meditative posture means to keep your head, neck and trunk straight. If you are sitting in the lotus posture and creating a hump in your back, that is not a correct posture. The posture that keeps your head, neck and trunk straight is the right posture.

Gently close your eyes and seal your lips. Between your chest and abdomen lies the diaphragm. Learn to use your diaphragm and form the habit of breathing with it so that its deep rhythmic movement becomes automatic. When you exhale let your diaphragm push in and help the lungs expel carbon dioxide or waste gases. When you have completely exhaled let your diaphragm help to create another space for fresh air. Exhale again and inhale again at least five to ten times. Your attention should be directed toward the diaphragmatic movement. See that you are not creating a pause. Your breath should be deep, smooth, silent and without jerks. It should be as deep as you can comfortably exhale and inhale. Watch the capacity of your lungs so you do not strain your lungs. There is no need to hurry. When you have done this for some time you can forget the diaphragmatic movement. Be aware that when you exhale you are exhaling air that is extraneous to your body, and the air you are inhaling is necessary for a healthy body and a sound mind.

You are now mentally observing the gentle flow of your breath. If your mind is running here and there, you will find that your breath has become irregular. Remember that the breath and the mind have a close relationship so they reflect each other. Any sharp or disturbing emotional thought can change the breath. As you begin to observe the breath you may notice that you are creating a pause at the beginning and the end of the exhalation and inhalation cycles. It is hard in the beginning not to allow any pause between the exhalation and inhalation. It needs practice and special effort.

Do not suggest anything to your mind. Relaxation is a spontaneous effect of this method. Quietness and stillness of the body without any strain are the important factors. The more your body becomes still, the more you will find joy.

The seat of your mind is your brain that is at the crown of your head. Now allow your mind to travel systematically downward beginning with your forehead. This is a mental process. Your eyes are closed. Then you come from your forehead to your eyebrows, eyelids, cheeks and mouth. Make sure your lips are closed as you exhale and inhale. Repeat. Exhale and inhale. Now let your awareness come down to your jaw. Locate any tension in the neck and throat region, then the shoulders, arms, wrists, hands and fingers. Exhale as though you are expelling all tension, inhale as though you are receiving vital energy from the cosmos. Your hands, wrists, arms and shoulders are now free of tension. Your mind again comes to the throat area and then to the chest. Exhale and inhale at least four times here. As you exhale, expel all your worries and anxieties. When you inhale, you are inhaling vital energy. You are filling the depth of your lungs with cosmic energy. Allow your mind to travel down to your abdomen, hips, thighs, knees, calf muscles, ankles, feet and toes. Exhale as though your whole body is exhaling; inhale as though your whole body is inhaling. Exhale and inhale again. Continue exhaling and inhaling as you gently lead the mind back up systematically to the crown of your head. Begin from the toes. Your toes have no tension. The ankles have no tension. Calf muscles, knees, hip joints, all have no tension. Exhale and inhale. Now, direct the mind along the vertebrae locating the tension in the spinal column. Gently come up, releasing the tension from the vertebrae until you reach the crown of your head.

Again let your mind be aware of the calm and serene flow of your breath. Breath and mind are twin laws of life. They interact, they react, they respond to each other. Let your mind make a gentle conscious effort to guide your breath so that it remains calm, deep and without any noise or jerks. Slowly and gently open your eyes.

Now, do not forget to repeat this process at least twice a day. That relaxation and the preliminary step toward meditation that you are seeking will soon be yours. Develop a practice. OM peace, peace, peace.

MEDITATION PRACTICUM NUMBER 4

Gently close your eyes and survey your body from head to toe. Your mind will tell you which part of the body has some tension. Where there is physical strain, you will find it is related to your mind and your emotions. Survey and relax every part of the body systematically from the toes up to the crown of your head. Attend to your breath after that. Push in your upper abdomen to help your diaphragm expel the carbon dioxide and used up gases. When you exhale, feel as though you are exhaling all your problems, worries and pains. When you inhale, inhale as though you are receiving vital energy from the atmosphere. And then do not think of breath and mind. Go beyond and observe your thinking process. A thought comes and goes away. Let it go.

Once you have learned not to identify with the thought patterns then you have to start the process of introspection, or inspecting within. Learn to be patient with yourself and persist in your efforts. Never give up or say you cannot train yourself. If you persist you will gradually expand your capacity. With the help of training, you can change the grooves of your mind and help yourself. Be vigilant. In this way you will find that the myriad of thoughts that are coming from the unconscious where you have stored many impressions from your daily life will not affect you. You are simply being a witness. During that time your mind, nervous system, muscles and all the tissues and cells will get perfect rest. Even if you cannot go beyond that, it's very healthy to sit still. Any method of meditation is helpful and healthy and very useful.

MEDITATION PRACTICUM NO. 5

Don't allow your mind to roam around, but gently direct your mind to a particular path. First, pay attention to the flow of your breath. Take five deep, even breaths, without creating any noise, jerk or pause in the breath. Observe the movement of the upper abdomen with the breath. Now, take the focus of the mind from the breath to the body. Be aware of your toes. From the tips of the toes systematically release all tension from your toes, feet, ankles, knees, hip joints, perineum, abdomen, chest, forearms, arms, chest, neck and face. Release all tension from the whole body. When you exhale the breath, exhale all tension and worries from the mind. Now, exhale slowly as though you are exhaling from the crown of your head to your toes. Then again inhale energy from the toes back to the crown of your head. On the next exhalation, exhale to the ankles and inhale from the ankles back to the crown of your head. Exhale to your knees and inhale from the knees to the crown of your head. Exhale to the perineum, and inhale from the perineum to the crown of your head. Exhale to the navel center and inhale from the navel to the crown of your head. Exhale to the space between the two breasts and inhale up to the crown of your head. Exhale to your throat center and inhale to the crown of your head. Now exhale to the bridge between the two nostrils. This is very important. Let your mind focus on the place between the two nostrils, asking your mind to allow the breath to flow freely through both nostrils. Follow the flow of breath between the bridge between the two nostrils and the crown of your head. You will find the breath has become very fine. Now exhale from the crown of your head down to the throat center.

Breathe deeply from the throat center to the crown of your head, exhaling down to the heart center. Again inhale to the crown of your head. Then exhale to the navel center, inhaling back to the crown of your head. Exhale to the perineum, and come back to the crown of your head.

Exhale to your knees, again come back to the crown of your head. Exhale to the ankles, inhale coming back to the crown of your head. Exhale to your toes, inhale from your toes to the crown of your head. Now let your whole body exhale and inhale. The movement of the breath is like a wave in the ocean. Inhalation is like a wave rising from the ocean; exhalation is like a wave going back to the ocean. Remember, the body is your grossest instrument, the breath is a subtler instrument and even subtler are the senses. The mind is your subtlest instrument. But you are not body, breath, senses and mind. Your essential nature is peace, happiness and wisdom. Now breathe gently to your fullest capacity.

INTERMEDIATE MEDITATION

Take your seat in a calm and quiet place, keeping your head, neck, and trunk straight. Do not strain yourself or over stretch. Let your hands rest steadily on your thighs or knees. Seal your teeth and lips gently. Gently push in the upper abdomen to contract your diaphragm as you exhale from your nostrils. When you inhale your upper abdomen should come out effortlessly and the diaphragm will also release. Repeat 10 to 15 times. See that your diaphragmatic movement is gentle and complete according to your comfortable capacity.

Now, focus your mind on the flow of the breath. Let your mind become aware that you are not creating any noise in the breath. You should make conscious effort to eliminate the pause between the inhalation and exhalation. Your breath is becoming calm, serene and deep. The more your mind is coordinated with the flow of the breath, the more you will experience an unusual joy.

Now let your mind focus on the bridge between the two nostrils. Here you can feel the breath coming in and going out. Let your mind be aware that both nostrils are flowing freely. If you find one of your nostrils is blocked or clogged, just meditate on that nostril and it will open up. Simple awareness will help you. With slight effort for a few days the mind will notice that both nostrils have started to flow freely because you have started to pay attention to the bridge between the two nostrils. When your mind has started to notice that both nostrils are inhaling and exhaling simultaneously, you will experience a state of joy. Then, the application of sushumna will lead the mind to a state of calmness. A joyous mind is necessary to make the mind one-pointed and inward.

Now, so far you are not remembering any mantra but you are just meditating on the bridge between the two nostrils. The more your body becomes calm and still, the more your muscles will become free from tension. You do not need to exert your lungs for want of extra oxygen. When the motion of lungs is regulated, the heart and involuntary systems are relaxed.

Now, let your mind focus on the center between the two eyebrows. Here you will have to be aware that you are not consciously trying to visualize anything, but just allow the mind to let go without any resistance. Remember that your mind has the habit to identify with the objects of the world or the objects of your thoughts. Try not to brood on any thoughts that are appearing before you. Witness the activities of your mind and if the mind is roaming around, gradually bring it back to the center between the two eyebrows. This center is called ajna chakra. Ajna chakra is a very important center that is the entrance to the city of life. It is the seat of the conscious mind during the waking state. Let your thought patterns flow without any interruption. Observe your thinking process, but do not allow your mind to be involved with it. Continue to focus your mind on the center between the two eyebrows. No object to meditate on is given at ajna chakra. It is a place of light that comes from within through your eyes. You will better understand if you put your fingers at the corners of the eyelids. If you do this, you'll find a glint of light coming from the side through your eyes. When you close your eyes this center is *divya chakshu*. Divya chakshu refers to the third eye that is a portal to intuitive wisdom and the higher levels of consciousness.

Now, be sensitive to the finer energy channels flowing along your spinal column. On your spinal column lay three channels. The channel in the center is called the centralis canalis and has within it the energy flow of sushumna. On both sides of your spinal columns are two ganglionated cords, the sympathetic and parasympathetic cords. The more you focus your mind on the central channel, the more your mind becomes sensitive and capable of being aware of these finer channels within.

Now, let your mind be aware of the vibrations of the perennial sound. The sound you hear along this channel is *so hum*. Your mind is flowing with the flow of the central channel to the root of your spinal column. When your mind is tuned to listen to the sound vibrations, inhale with the sound *so* up to the crown of your head; and exhale with the sound *hum* down to the root of your spinal column. *So hum* is a universal sound that means "that I am." *So* means "that," *hum* means "this." At the root of your spinal column lies the primal, dormant force of consciousness that is called kundalini. Kundalini awakening is not what you think it is. It means the capacity to fathom many levels of consciousness, but first you have to develop body awareness. When you awaken this source you can experience all the levels of consciousness systematically.

Silently meditate on the sound vibrations coming from your spinal cord *so....hum....* Feel as though your mind is inhaling and exhaling through your spinal column. With the exhalation repeat the sound *hum* down to the root of the spinal column to awaken the primal force. Then inhale to the crown of your head while repeating the sound *so* to lead that primal force to the highest of your chakras, the crown chakra or sahasrara chakra.

Now, again pay attention to the center between the two eyebrows and remember the mantra your teacher has given to you. Let your mind be focused on the sound vibrations of your mantra. Your teeth should be sealed and your tongue should not move. When you listen to the sound of your mantra, you may find your attention sometimes slipping as you may begin to feel tired. When this happens you should stop and try again later. You should remember your mantra in a way so that your mind follows the sound of the mantra. This method will still the body, free tension from the muscles and relax the mind. You should also form the habit of remembering your mantra while doing your duties. Your mantra can be your companion wherever you go.

Remember that you have a body, which is your gross instrument. Your breath and your senses are your subtle instruments and your mind is your finest instrument. But you are not your body, breath, senses or mind. You are seated beyond your body, breath, senses and mind in a calm and quiet chamber within. Exhale all anxiety, problems, stress and strain; inhale vital force and energy. Allow your breath to become smooth, calm and serene. You are like an eternal wave of bliss in the vast space, undisturbed and fearless. You are a child of eternity. Now, determine that you will no longer identify with your mind and its objects. Be constantly aware of the center of consciousness as you perform your duties, skillfully and selflessly. Exhale and inhale again.

OM shanti, shanti, shanti.
Peace, peace, peace.

ADVANCED MEDITATION

My way of using the mantra is different from yours. I sit down, and I see my whole being listening to the mantra. I do not remember the mantra mentally, because then the mind repeats many things. Instead,

I make my whole being an ear to listen to the mantra, and it is coming from all over.

This will not happen to you immediately in meditation. Only after you have attained or accomplished something will this happen. Then, even if you decide that you do not want to remember the mantra, it is not possible. Finally, even the mantra does not exist, but the purpose for which you are repeating the mantra is there. The mantra might still be there but as an experience that overwhelms your whole being, and it is not separate from you.

COMING OUT OF MEDITATION

What you should do after meditation, and the question of how you should continue meditation during the whole day are also very important. You are taught to prepare for meditation, but you are not taught how to come out of meditation. You should come out of meditation with the same consciousness you have attained during meditation. During that time you are close to the reality. As time passes, you may grow far away from the reality. Determine that you will always have the consciousness and awareness you have during meditation, no matter where you go. In this way, constant consciousness and awareness will lead to wisdom and give you freedom from all misery and bondage. Nothing should disturb you. Learn to think with clarity of mind and do not brood or worry.

OM peace, peace, peace.

KUNDALINI

INTOXICATION

Between mind and soul lies a force called kundalini shakti, which is a deeper, direct power of the individual soul or center of consciousness. It is symbolized as a resting serpent at the root of the spinal column and is the dormant support of the entire body and all its pranic energies. KUNDALINI IS THE DIVINE FORCE IN THE HUMAN BODY. In other words, all the energy of the entire body evolves from the kundalini shakti. That shakti powerhouse has come from the individual soul. In Sanskrit, kundalini is called Devatma shakti. Devatma consists of two words: *deva* and *atma*. *Deva* means "bright being," *atma* means "bright being within you." Atma is Atman, the individual or cosmic soul. The word *soul* in Sanskrit is atma, individual soul is jivatma and cosmic soul is Paramatma. That Atman is the eternal center of consciousness within you. The individual soul functions with the help of Devatma shakti. *Shakti* means "power."

Even though the word *kundalini* is frequently used, it is a very secretive word according to the highest order of yoga and other branches of Indian, Tibetan and Chinese philosophies. It is not properly understood, even in India or by great scholars, because it is subject to direct experience. There are several meanings of the Sanskrit term *kundalini*. *Kunda* means "bowl of fire;" *lini* means "that which dwells in the bowl of fire." *Kundala* means "that which is coiled." One who dwells in a cave is also called *kundalini*. According to tantric philosophy and mythology, the dormant force that supports the universe is symbolized by a serpent-like coiled up energy. Kunda is the bowl of fire and the coiled energy is the serpent fire, the kundalini shakti. The closest translation of the word kundalini in the English language is *consciousness* or *awareness*.

Kundalini is the finest form of energy that individuals have. Very little of this kundalini energy is activated and expressed in the functioning of the chakras or the nadis. Instead, in most human beings, the vast unknown power of kundalini energy simply lies latent and unexpressed. However, in every era and civilization there have been those who somehow, consciously or unconsciously, have tapped into some part of this infinite reservoir of energy. Those individuals have been the geniuses and dynamic forces throughout human history.

Kundalini energy is said to rest at the base of the spine in the human body at muladhara, the lowest chakra. Here there is a cavity where that fire remains in a dormant or sleeping state. However, kundalini's real home is swadhishthana chakra, "HER OWN ABODE." She sleeps at the root chakra because she is intoxicated from taking the nectar *(amrita)* that drips from the *Brahmakhanda,* the ocean of nectar from where the nectar is continuously dripping from within the head, thus depriving the individual of what should be theirs. Even with all the ability, potential and knowledge of a human being, as long as kundalini is dormant, jiva will remain brute-like and unable to expand to universal consciousness. If you prevent her from taking that nectar, she awakens.

THE CHAKRAS AND KUNDALINI

The study of the chakras is very intriguing and profound. However, as with the concept of kundalini, much of what is said or written about the chakras is inaccurate, distorted or misleading. A complete and accurate description of the system of the chakras would require another book, and even then, one could not really understand the chakras until their influence was directly experienced.

The knowledge of the chakras is not even a hundred years old in the West. The science of the chakras has been explained in the Book of Revelation, both in Jewish and Christian literature. Buddhism and Hinduism also bank on the subtle knowledge of the chakras. There are seven main chakras: muladhara, swadhishthana, manipura, anahata, vishuddha, ajna and sahasrara. Anahata chakra divides the two hemispheres. Here two triangles meet to form a six-pointed star. One triangle flows downwards, and the other flows upwards. The upward flowing triangle represents the ascending force; and the downward flowing triangle is the descending force. The ascending force comes from sincere human effort. The descending force is grace. They meet at anahata chakra. By contemplating and concentrating on anahata chakra, you can have control over your emotions and thus experience perfect equilibrium and tranquillity.

According to tantric texts, it is very necessary for a student of this path to have a clear and comprehensive knowledge of the chakras before they start to practise the process of awakening the kundalini. Yoga science is very complex and extensive. It includes the science of the body and knowledge of the nervous system and subtler energy levels that govern bodily functions. In addition, careful study of the mind, its modifications, and all states of consciousness, as well as the philosophy of the universe and human relationships are included. Tantra philosophy integrates all these various levels of knowledge and energy. All the diverse areas of science, psychology and philosophy are integrated in tantra philosophy, and all facets of the individual can be coordinated by means of sincere efforts. By learning to explore the inner world, thoughts and emotions, the student attempts to unveil all the mysteries of the various levels of life and experiments with experiencing different aspects of their being and different reactions of the world.

The energy of shakti is organized around the seven chakras, which are like intense vortices of energy. The student of tantric yoga studies these centers, their nature and their interrelationships. The more they understand the various psychological and philosophical concepts of the chakras, the more they find it necessary to know all the levels within the framework of the physical body.

The chakras are said to be arranged along the midline of the body, in correspondence with the spinal column, from the base of the spine to the crown of the head. The chakras energize, control and influence regions of the body, although they themselves cannot be perceived on the physical level. While the chakras are not physical centers, they definitely affect the physical body, each having a specific area of correspondence.

Manifestation of the cosmic force is expressed through these centers. Each center has its particular frame of reference through which the individual experiences the world. Kundalini manifests in the form of each center. For example, when mind and energy are expressed through the heart or fourth chakra, one becomes loving and is able to control emotional energy. Similarly, when mind and energy are predominantly expressed through the second chakra, one is preoccupied with thoughts of sexuality.

The chakras also determine the level of consciousness in a human being. Energy is usually focused predominantly in one chakra, with less energy available in the other centers. The differences between how this energy is focused account for differences in personality, and level of consciousness. The grossest level of energy is at the base, and then it starts to become subtler and finer until you reach the subtlest energy in sahasrara. Of the seven chakras, the lowest six are the easiest to describe. The first two chakras—the first at the base of the spine, and the second at the genital area—reflect the lowest level of consciousness and the most primitive ways of experiencing the world. These chakras are related to the instincts for physical survival and preservation of the species. From a spiritual point of view, these chakras and their energy have a quality of heaviness, inertia and ignorance of pure consciousness. When these chakras predominate, there is little awareness of, or interest in, higher spiritual evolution.

The next two chakras, located at the navel and heart centers, create more energy, movement and active involvement. They relate to issues of autonomy, self-control, power and the sense of self, as well as to the ability to love and empathize with others. These two chakras reflect somewhat more evolved "human" issues, as opposed to the more primitive and instinctive "animal" issues of the first two chakras.

The two chakras located at the throat and brow regions encompass a more highly evolved level of consciousness. Their influence is one of creativity, serenity, intuition and wisdom. Although there are other subtle centers above the brow center, the final center is located at the crown of the head, and is said to be the final abode of consciousness within the individual. Usually, a human being's energy is divided, with the energy of pure translucent consciousness at the crown of the head, while the dormant power of kundalini shakti rests or sleeps at the base of the spine.

PREPARATION FOR AWAKENING THE KUNDALINI

In order to awaken the kundalini, the sincere and motivated student must first prepare themself on all levels. Concrete and profound practice is needed. You should know what you are doing, otherwise you will be wasting your time and it could be dangerous. You have to understand you are doing these practices to awaken the sleeping power. Otherwise, you will remain a brute who can function in the external world but not within.

It is important for the student to be aware that awakening the kundalini generally is attained only after prolonged study, self-purification and preparation that includes basic practices, such as learning how to maintain a healthy body and to control mind, action and speech. The student may also observe silence and other physical and mental disciplines. It is most important that a student should be steady and systematic in their practice and should not initiate rash, intense practices or indulge in emotional outbursts. In this way, the student will gradually and steadily expand their capacity and bring about rapid, consistent progress. When the student makes prolonged, sincere efforts, they raise the ascending force, and then the descending force called grace *(kripa)* will also dawn.

First, the physical body needs to be purified and strengthened, especially through practices such as hatha yoga, breathing exercises and maintaining a correct diet. If the teacher does not teach anything but physical postures in hatha yoga, after some time the student will notice the breath is creating problems. The practice of hatha yoga helps to create awareness of your breathing patterns. When you start to understand how your breath and body can work harmoniously together, then you want to know more about the mind. Next, you will want to go beyond mind and tap into the unconscious mind. This is called self-education or self-training. You will not get this experience from reading books. Experience should become your guide. Otherwise, you will not be satisfied.

On the mental and emotional levels, too, the sincere student must prepare themselves by learning the basic practices of yoga required to balance the emotions, coordinate the mind and channel the higher energy involved. Such preparation is crucial because a sudden increase of this latent power can disorient and disrupt the overall functioning of a person who has not yet become calm, balanced and able to integrate the higher energy levels. Even on the mere physical level, a sudden increase and release of kundalini energy can cause disturbances or imbalance. This is like a situation in which a high voltage electrical current is channeled through a weak and inadequate wiring system. Only when the physical system is strong, balanced and prepared, can it safely assimilate the energy of kundalini. Because of this, authentic teachers never teach advanced practices for the awakening of kundalini to unprepared students but instead use the methods of yoga to train students to prepare themselves. It is this period of preparation for the awakening of the kundalini that is the most important in the entire training process. Now, if a teacher has tilled the land, they will sow the seeds. But if a teacher is a fool and does not know—by chance they got the seeds from their guru—they will sow the seeds on untilled land. The duty of the teacher is to prepare you first, to till the land and then to sow the seeds. It is your duty to see that the seeds grow.

The system of yoga includes several techniques that are specifically intended to help prepare the student. These include the following:

1) Hatha yoga strengthens the body and helps to prepare it for the increase in energy. Traditionally, hatha yoga is used in combination with purificatory processes, such as washes that cleanse and refine the physical body and nervous system.

2) Hatha yoga with breathing exercises make up one unit. Breathing exercises and pranayama are the finest of all exercises. Physical exercise with relaxation exercises comprise another unit. Pranayama allows the student to learn how to channel the pranic energy and eventually raise the kundalini. Pranayama exercises also affect the balance of the nervous system and help to create a calm, quiet mind. The mind is generally preoccupied with the stimulation it receives from the external world via the senses, but once this energy is focused within, the student is able to alter the mind's tendency to be scattered. The breathing exercises help the student to raise and channel energy through the central pathway, sushumna. In this manner, kundalini is drawn upwards.

Editor's note: Once I asked Swamiji if the practice of pranayama leads to the control of the five pranas, he replied, "Why only the five pranas? It leads to control of the whole pranic sheath and the flow of energy through all 72,000 nadis."

3) Concentration and meditation practices on certain chakras help to shift consciousness from the body and its physical functions, to an inner state. Meditation on a chakra may help to raise kundalini to that chakra.

4) Practices of higher tantra involve physical and mental celibacy. This energy is elevated to a higher level by meditating on the union of Shiva and Shakti within.

5) Kundalini can also be awakened by those who raise their energy through intellectual study of philosophical scriptures, or by those who are intensely devotional.

HOW TO AWAKEN THE KUNDALINI

There are also some crude methods for awakening the kundalini. I could raise your kundalini in one second's time whether you were prepared or not. But then you would faint. You would go through all the signs of kundalini awakening but when you wake up again the kundalini would have returned to muladhara where she remains asleep. Some people accidentally come in touch with the kundalini, and when it awakens in this manner, it could be painful. This is a very scientific method of awakening the sleeping energy, the primal force that is in the reservoir in the human body. Many of you have that little bit. Sometimes she awakens and you become very creative. For example, you may start to write poems or you may start to dance very well. Any person who is above average such as artists, writers and doctors, it is because of the effect of the energy of the kundalini.

There is one great beauty in the path of awakening the kundalini. If you have awakened your kundalini in this lifetime and then you leave your body, in the next lifetime you will start from where you have left off. You don't have to start over from the beginning. KUNDALINI PRACTICE IS MUCH DEEPER THAN MEDITATION.

HATHA YOGA AND AWAKENING THE KUNDALINI

Asanas and the study of mudras and cleansings come under the domain of physical exercises, but they are only part of the vast system of hatha yoga. If you limit hatha yoga to exercises, you are misusing the word. First, you should understand the two symbols *ha* and *tha*. You are directly receiving prana through your two nostrils. The symbol of one prana is *ha,* and the symbol of the other is *tha.* Hatha yoga is a science that is complete in itself. The highest and subtlest form of this science is called awakening the kundalini. YOU CANNOT UNDERSTAND THE SPIRITUAL ASPECT OF HATHA IF YOU DO NOT UNDERSTAND THE KUNDALINI.

According to hatha yoga there are several ways to awaken the kundalini. One way is by doing *mudras* (gestures). This is body language. You can easily know the nature of a person if you understand body language. According to yoga, *body language* means "the study of mudras," of which there are several hundred forms. For example, in *maha mudra,* the left heel is placed at the root of the spinal cord. The right foot is caught hold of by the toe and the nose is put on the knee. You stay in that position for three hours.

Another method suggested is *shirsasana,* the headstand. I think that is more symbolic and should not be taken literally. If you literally stand on your head, it is a good exercise, but you cannot stand the whole day on your head; and even if you were able to do this your life would be useless. Instead, you should stand within your center, the real head within you, atma. You are taught to do the headstand so that you can stand on your own two feet. If you cannot do the headstand, it is not due to any physical problem. You fall because you have no confidence and no control. I tell students to sit down and first do the headstand mentally. According to hatha yoga, your head is the center of consciousness of the soul. To stand on your head means you should have self-confidence and be aware of the center of consciousness. That is the actual headstand. It is said in the manuals that if you remain in the headstand for three hours, the kundalini will be awakened. Actually, there is no need to do this. You can awaken the kundalini in two minutes, but you have to be prepared for that. There is a particular spot you have to hit with the heel, and after that you will no longer be using your senses. You have a vision where you find yourself expanding and you come in touch with a chemical substance in your body that is very intoxicating and puts you into very deep sleep. According to the yoga manuals, if you have insomnia and cannot sleep it is because certain glands are not secreting properly. With the help of certain exercises you can improve the functioning of those sleep glands.

KHECHARI MUDRA

Yogis know how to drink the nectar that kundalini shakti has been taking. According to hatha yoga, by applying *khechari* mudra (the tongue mudra), the yogi can awaken the kundalini. *Kha* means "space," or "sky;" *chari* means "tongue, tip of the tongue." *Khechari* means "one who travels in the sky." Every fountain can give you water to quench your thirst, but only this fountain can give you the nectar that can make you immortal and give you intuitive knowledge. This method is not used in tantra and other branches of yoga. When the tip of the tongue is inserted in the space behind the palate, then you start to travel in that sky. In khechari mudra you put the tip of the tongue inward and upward toward the palate and gently touch it. From there the nectar you receive will have one of two tastes: the taste of mother's milk *(amrit kala)* or the taste of ghee *(swalp kala)*. It is not your choice which taste you acquire from there; it depends on your potentiality. Those who receive amrit kala become like Shankaracharya, very slim and gentle, like a beautiful woman. On the other hand, those who receive swalp kala become so strong they could fight with an elephant or a tiger. Jesus Christ was a very strong person, physically and mentally both. A spiritual person is very strong because their mind remains one-pointed. Mental equilibrium and physical tranquillity can do immense wonders in the world.

In addition, with the help of prana through rhythmic breathing you can awaken the fire. The theme of fire as facilitator of purification is repeated throughout the Yoga Sutras. When a smith uses the bellows, the fire remains active. If he doesn't use the bellows, a layer of ashes comes. If you pay attention toward the sensation of the flow and the overlapping of the channels of energy within you, you can go to the root of the spinal cord with your mind and become aware of that sleeping fire. Some people are sensitive and can easily do this, and some are not, but they can be brought to sensitivity. If you learn to be very sensitive, you can sense all things around you. That is why Paramahamsa Ramakrishna used to say he would feel pin pricks when a bad person would come to him, and when a good person would come, he would feel good vibes. You have lost that sensitivity. Do not misunderstand that to create sensitivity does not mean to become sensual.

My kung fu teacher was blind and older than 90 years of age. I have never seen such a calm and strong person in my life. Once while we were walking he told me to pick up a stone and throw it at him. I thought he would surely die if I did that. He insisted I should do it to examine his alertness. I told him I was very strong and he might die if I threw a stone at him. He said, "Why do you not show me your strength then?" Another day we were walking side by side and I suddenly moved my wrist with the intention to hit him. He caught hold of me abruptly and continued to walk as though nothing had happened. I examined him three or four times in this way, and he never failed to impress me with his level of sensitivity. He could sense my movement through its vibrations. Though he could not see, he was very sensitive to the environment and any vibrations.

SIDDHASANA

There are two sets of postures in hatha yoga—cultural and meditative. The word *posture* does not come from exercise. Human beings make many postures. If you do yoga postures it will make you more aware of balance. The moment you lose your balance, you fall down. The uniqueness of hatha yoga is that in hatha yoga you are training your mind through your body. Other exercises do not make you aware of your mind.

When yogis sit in meditation, they use a meditative posture called siddhasana (accomplished pose). With the help of siddhasana and agni sara, you can awaken the kundalini. Siddhasana is used to help control sexual desire. This particular pose directly affects muladhara and the sacral plexus, which in turn immediately affect the ductless glands, the testes and the ovaries. These glands are responsible for controlling hormonal balance of that particular area. A person who sits in this pose for a long time will find thoughts of sex disturb less frequently. Otherwise, some people don't have that control and they think of sex all the time. Others may be motivated by overeating or sleeping all the time. You will see that one of the urges is prominent in different individuals. All these urges can be cultured and brought under control.

It is helpful for those who want to meditate and lead a single life to practise siddhasana often, but it should not be done more than a half hour at a time by one who lives in the world. A renunciant should practise it more than two hours and five minutes. Then he is cut off from his motor system, as all the lower extremities are controlled by this particular posture. After doing two and a half hours of this posture you are cut off from pain, though when you leave this posture you are back to normal.

AGNI SARA

In hatha yoga there is one exercise, agni sara, that is used for that particular agni that functions in the solar plexus and helps with your digestion. The vagus nerve also facilitates digestion. When you do agni sara you are also helping to regulate the motion of your lungs. It takes three or four months to perfect and develop control over the abdominal muscles. Do not push them out; just let them come out, otherwise you will have a bulging tummy. When you take the abdomen in you use force but when you take it out you do not. This will also help to increase the gastric juices.

AGNI SARA PRACTICUM

Agni sara and the stomach lift are two entirely different things. The abdominal lift prepares your abdomen to do agni sara, and agni sara prepares you to activate your solar system. To begin with, you should do it twenty-five times. Then gradually work up to a hundred times at least.

In agni sara you pull in above the public bone, and then the abdominal contents roll up toward the chest cavity after you pull up.

First, you should practise the stomach lift for one or two months so your abdominal muscles will become more supple. Then, when your abdominal muscles become supple, you draw in right from the pelvis, as though something is rolling up. And then relax but don't force.

In accordance with diaphragmatic breathing, when you practise agni sara, one rule is to be applied from the very beginning. When you push in your abdomen, you have to exhale; and when you relax and allow the abdomen to come out, you have to inhale. Don't force the abdomen to come out when you inhale. Force should be used only when you exhale, not in inhalation. In this way the diaphragm presses against your lungs and it becomes easy for you to exhale. That regulates the motion of your lungs and helps the motion to expel the carbon dioxide and used up gases.

The ideal time it takes to do one agni sara is according to your capacity. My capacity differs from your capacity, so the ideal time also differs. Perhaps I have practised a long breath, and you have not. So, the ideal time goes according to the length of each breath within your individual capacity. In agni sara you should not breathe quickly or you will not be able to draw in the whole abdomen as required.

You can do the stomach lift faster, but in agni sara you cannot complete the entire roll if you try to do more than one lift per breath. Sometimes even one breath is not sufficient to complete the entire roll. You have to coordinate your breath and the muscle pull.

You can also do agni sara on a chair. Begin by putting your hands on the abdomen. On exhaling push your abdomen in as far as you can. Then gently relax your hands and allow the abdomen to come out as you inhale naturally.

---

the awakening

The main goal of meditation is to awaken the kundalini and lead it to the highest state of consciousness. By awakening the kundalini shakti, you will be with the eternal and free from all anxiety, misery and pain. As long as shakti remains dormant and coiled, the human being remains a brute because they are not consciously taking that nectar. With the help of mantras, the mind can go to that sleeping force and awaken it. Then it travels upward passing through the chakras, the seven levels of consciousness. When the kundalini passes through the chakras, the chakras change. The descriptions of the chakras you are familiar with are referring to the chakras before kundalini has passed through them.

Long before physics, yoga described seven levels of consciousness. The Roman Bible describes seven words, while in music there are seven key notes, no matter which music you study. This comes from the music that goes on within you. In physics, it is said there are seven spheres in the universe and the energy moves in a different pattern from one sphere to another. Take the example of electricity. The electrons move in a certain direction, and not randomly or in an opposite way. They move according to a pattern or law and not contrary to it. It is a well understood law in physics that all protons move toward the center. But on this level, the energy is gross. On subtler levels the energy becomes finer and finer until it finds its center. Just as there is a place of power in a city or country, one's center is the place that supplies energy to the whole being. That is why it is said, *Deho devalaya prokta jivo deva sanantan:* This body is like a temple, and THE INNER DWELLER IS THE ETERNAL ONE, THAT WHO IS.

PATHWAY OF THE KUNDALINI

When a yogi consciously takes that nectar, thus depriving the kundalini shakti, then there is some movement at the base of the spinal cord as the kundalini becomes aroused. No longer intoxicated, she becomes very angry and fierce with all her seven tongues out and immediately begins to search for that nectar. There are three main tubes along the spinal column. The central tube is the centralis canalis, and on both sides are the ganglionated cords. Inside this centralis canalis there is an energy channel, the *brahmani.* It is like a tube within a tube, *chitrani* and then brahmani. It is called brahmani because if you tap that channel you can easily go to the Brahman rudra. Although there are three channels leading to this, the kundalini shakti wakes up and with all her fierce anxiety pushes herself through the finest channel, sushumna. First, she goes to her own abode, swadhishthana chakra, then to the next chakra, manipura and continues upward, piercing all the chakra centers to finally reach sahasrara where she meets her beloved.

BHUTA SHUDDHI

THE FOLLOWING PRACTICE OF BHUTA SHUDDHI IS REPRODUCED HERE WITH MINOR CHANGES FROM THE WEBSITE SWAMIJ.COM WITH PERMISSION FROM THE AUTHOR, SWAMI JNANESHWARA BHARATI.

Chakra Meditation
Bhuta Shuddhi
Purifying the Five Elements
by Swami Jnaneshwara Bharati
SwamiJ.com

Method of Practicing Chakra Meditation—
Bhuta Shuddhi

Bhuta Shuddhi is an ancient chakra meditation of yoga and tantra practice through which the five elements (bhutas) are balanced or purified (shuddhi). Bhuta refers to the past, and shuddhi refers to purifying that past, or the samskaras that operate in conjunction with the five elements. This is a very useful practice, whether you think of it as preparation for kundalini awakening, or simply as a practice for feeling balanced, centered or tranquil,

For the chakra meditation of bhuta shuddhi, it is necessary to understand how the five elements relate to the chakras. The five bhutas are the five elements: earth, water, fire, air and space, and they operate in

Chakra	Element	Mantra	Karmen-driya	Jnanendriya
7	(consciousness)	Silence	(consciousness)	(consciousness)
6	(mind)	OM	(mind)	(mind)
5	space	Ham*	speaking	hearing
4	air	Yam*	grasping / holding	touching
3	fire	Ram*	moving	seeing
2	water	Vam*	procreating	tasting
1	earth	Lam*	eliminating	smelling

*Pronounced like "Tom," "Mom," or "CD-ROM"

conjunction with the lower five chakras. At a subtler level they are called *tanmatras*, which are part of the tattvas, or subtle constituents). The sixth chakra is of mind, and is beyond or prior to the bursting forth of space, air, fire, water, and finally earth. Consciousness itself is prior to, or the source of manifestation of mind, and is the seventh chakra.

Each chakra has a bija mantra associated with it. You might enjoy simply breathing up and down the sushumna channel, the subtle spine, either with OM going up and down, or *so hum*, with *so* going up to the crown and *hum* going down to the base of the spine.

The five elements align with and operate from the five lower chakras, along with the ten indriyas and a seed mantra for each. In systematic chakra meditation, you progressively move attention through the chakras, along with awareness of the nature of each chakra.

There may be many methods of purifying the five elements, ranging from meditative practices, including yoga nidra, to various forms of ritualistic practices. With some reflection it makes sense how it is that many practices might have such an effect. Bhuta shuddhi works directly with attention on the chakras, balancing the subtle forces of the five elements through the use of the bija (seed) mantras of the chakras.

Before doing the bhuta shuddhi practice itself, it is useful to do some stretches or hatha asanas followed by some form of physical relaxation exercise, such as a complete relaxation. This helps prepare the mind to be able to focus on the chakras.

Bhuta shuddhi: Sequentially move through the chakras in the following sequence. As you read this, please keep in mind that reading about the practice is more difficult than doing the practice. The descriptions are lengthy, but the practices are actually straightforward and simple.

1. Muladhara Chakra Meditation: Bring your attention to the perineum, the flat space between the anus and the genital area. Take several seconds to allow your attention to find the space and to get settled into it. Allow the mantra LAM to arise repeatedly in your mind field, silently. Allow it to repeat at its own natural speed. You may find that it comes five to ten times and then wants to pause, or you might find it wants to come continuously. If it pauses, allow it to return in its own time. The mantra may move quickly or slowly. In any case, keep your attention on that space; this is

very important. That space might be tiny, such as a pinpoint, or it might be several inches across. Follow your own inclination about the size of the space. Allow your mind to naturally be aware of earth, solidity or form. That awareness may come a little or a lot; either way is okay. Allow to come through your mind field the awareness of the karmendriya of elimination and the jnanendriya of smell. Gradually it will become clearer how it is that the indriyas operate from these centers, along with the five elements. You may or may not also find that colors and sounds naturally come to the inner field of mind.

2. Swadhishthana Chakra Meditation: When you move your attention upward toward the second chakra, be mindful of the transition, of the motion of attention and the nature of the shift of energetic, emotional and mental experience. Allow your attention to naturally find the location of the second chakra. Your own attention will find and settle into that space. It is important to note that the actual chakra is in the back, along the subtle spinal energy channel, sushumna. Allow the attention to rest where it naturally falls. Gradually, attention will find this central stream running up and down through all of the chakras. Sushumna is actually subtler than the chakras. Allow the mantra VAM to arise and repeat itself at its own speed, coming and going naturally. Hold your attention in the space, whether a pinpoint or a few inches across. Allow the awareness of water to arise, and come to see what this has to do to allow the forms of flow or fluidity, whether relating to energy, physical, emotional or mental. Explore the awareness of the karmendriya of procreation and the jnanendriya of tasting. Again, colors or sounds may or may not come and go.

3. Manipura Chakra Meditation: Be aware of the transition as you move to the third chakra at the navel center, which is also actually along the sushumna

channel. Allow the mantra RAM to arise and repeat itself, at its natural pace. Keep your attention in the space at whatever size you experience. Be aware of the element of fire, and the many ways in which it operates throughout the gross and subtle body from this center. Be aware of the karmendriya of motion and how motion itself happens in so many physical, energetic and mental ways. Be aware of the jnanendriya of seeing, which you will easily see as related to fire and motion. Colors and sounds may or may not come and go.

4. Anahata Chakra Meditation: Observe the transition as you move your attention to the fourth chakra, the space between the two breasts. Allow attention to become well seated there, and then remember the vibration of the mantra YAM, allowing it to repeat at its own pace, while being mindful of the feeling it generates. Be aware of the element of air, and notice how that feels with the mantra. Notice how the element of air relates to the karmendriya of holding or grasping, whether physically, energetically, mentally or emotionally. Observe how these relate to the jnanendriya of touching, and how that touching is very subtle in addition to being a physical phenomenon. Colors and sounds may come and go.

5. Vishuddha Chakra Meditation: Bring your attention to the space at the throat, the fifth chakra, which is the point of emergence of space, which allows air, fire, water and earth to then emerge. In that space, be aware of the nature of space itself, allowing the mantra HAM to arise and repeat itself, reverberating many times through the seemingly empty space in the inner world, a space that is really not empty but is of potential. Awareness of the karmendriya of speech (actually, communication of any subtle form) is allowed to be there, experiencing how that vibrates through space. The jnanendriya of hearing is allowed to come, also seeing how it naturally aligns with

space, speech and the vibration of mantra. Notice the fine, subtle feelings that come with the experience. Colors or sounds are allowed to come and go, if they happen to arise.

6. Ajna Chakra Meditation: Gently, with full awareness, transition awareness to the seat of the mind at the space between the eyebrows, ajna chakra. Allow the mantra OM to arise and repeat itself, over and over, as slow waves of mantra, or as vibrations repeating so fast that the many OMs merge into a continuous vibration. Be aware of how mind has no elements, but is the source out of which space, air, fire, water and earth emerge. Be aware of how this space, mind itself, does no actions, but is the driving force of all of the karmendriyas of speech, holding, moving, procreating and eliminating. Be aware of how mind has no senses itself, but is the recipient of all of the information coming from hearing, touching, seeing, tasting and smelling, whether the source of this input is the sensations from the external world coming through the physical instruments, or coming from the inner world of memories or subtle experiences presenting on the mental screen through the subtle senses. Gradually, come to see how OM mantra is experienced as the source or map of manifestation itself. Many senses, images, or impressions may come and go, but they are let go, as attention rests in the knowing beyond all senses, in the ajna chakra and the vibration of OM.

7. Sahasrara Chakra Meditation: Allow attention to move to the crown chakra, which has no element (bhutas), no cognitive sense (jnanendriyas), no active means of expression (karmendriyas), as it is the doorway to pure consciousness itself. Experience how this is the source out of which mind emerges, after which emerge the five elements, the five cognitive senses and the five means of expression. The "mantra" in its subtler, silent form is that silence out

of which the rest have emerged. It is experienced as the silence after a single OM, merging into objectless, senseless awareness. Allow attention to rest in that pure stillness, the emptiness that is not empty, which contains and is the pure potential for manifestation, which has not manifested.

8. Ajna Chakra Meditation: Briefly bring your attention back to the sixth chakra, allowing the vibration of OM to return, which starts the journey of attention back into the body and the external world. A few seconds, or maybe a minute should be comfortable, though it may be longer if you wish.

9. Vishuddha Chakra Meditation: Bring your attention down to the fifth chakra, the throat, remembering HAM, as you enter into the realm of space, hearing, and speaking. Again, a few seconds or a minute is good.

10. Anahata Chakra Meditation: Transition to the fourth chakra, the spiritual heart, as you allow the mantra YAM to arise, remembering the element of air. Awareness of holding and touching may or may not arise.

11. Manipura Chakra Meditation: Be aware of the third chakra, the navel center, and the vibration of RAM, along with the element of fire, with awareness of motion and seeing coming or not coming.

12. Swadhishthana Chakra Meditation: Bring your attention to the second chakra, and allow the vibration of the mantra VAM to arise and repeat itself, remembering the element of water, with awareness of procreation and tasting coming or not coming.

13. Muladhara Chakra Meditation: Transition attention back to the first chakra, at the perineum, allowing the mantra LAM to come.

When first practicing bhuta shuddhi, it can seem confusing to keep track of mantras, elements, senses and actions. To make it easy, the two keys to emphasize initially are: 1) keeping your attention in the space, and 2) remembering the vibration of each mantra. It won't take very long to memorize which mantra goes with which chakra. Then allow the rest to gradually come in time. Both the balancing of the elements and chakras and the many insights will come over time with practice.

After the Practice: After the bhuta shuddhi practice itself, it is best to do some more meditation practice, since mind is now quite prepared. One good thing to do first is to practice the spinal breath where you bring your attention upward to the crown with inhalation and then follow the stream of the subtle spinal energy down to the first chakra with exhalation. This is nicely done with the so hum mantra where you inhale up with *soooo* and exhale down with *hummm*. This can then be followed by your regular meditation, allowing your attention to rest in only one of the chakras, the one where you regularly place attention during meditation or the place that feels the most comfortable.

SIGNS OF KUNDALINI AWAKENING

In modern times, many dramatic phenomena that are attributed to the awakening of kundalini are actually the result of nervous or emotional releases, rather than higher spiritual experiences. Certainly, unusual spiritual experiences can take place, but in the present day when there is such a level of misunderstanding, sensationalism and exploitation of the term *kundalini,* it is important to differentiate genuine from false experiences. Many people who are not physically, mentally or emotionally balanced attribute their experiences to some higher energy, rather than to other imbalances or difficulties. Some people use the kundalini only for worldly gains, attainments and enjoyment. But the authentic practice of yoga involves awakening the kundalini shakti and leading her systematically through the chakras to the crown chakra. When this takes place, the union of Shiva (pure consciousness) and Shakti occurs, and the individual becomes fully conscious. Then, one attains the highest state of samadhi. This state is the ultimate goal of yoga practice, but few achieve it.

What the yogis do to awaken her is to uncoil this force and lead it upward through sushumna, the finest channel in you that leads to the highest abode where her beloved resides. This is easily accomplished by yogis and devotees of Shri Vidya. More commonly, the student of yoga may awaken kundalini shakti and lead her only part of the way to the crown chakra. When this transformation takes place, and the individual activates some of this infinite potential, we say their kundalini has awakened. This usually takes place gradually, with small bursts of energy and shifts in consciousness, although sometimes such awakenings are sudden and intense. Such a great person whose kundalini is awakened knows the ultimate reality and thus has the gift of knowing that which is beyond time, space and causation. As an individual you can know the entire mystery of the universe, qualitatively speaking. However, a person who claims to know everything does not necessarily know truth.

SHAKTIPAT

Usually, the student practises several steps concurrently. For example, they may be doing asanas and breathing practices, as well as meditating on a mantra. As the student evolves and becomes skilled at managing and becoming more aware of increasingly finer energies, they may also be given other advanced practices. Eventually, these practices may lead to a step in which the teacher provides a higher initiation by sharing some of their own energy. However, even for this to take place, the student must already have refined and purified their body, mind and personality so they can respond to the teacher's assistance. This higher initiation is called *shaktipat*, and when it occurs, the student's consciousness is elevated to a higher level that is joyful, transcendent and serene. This state may last for various periods of time, but the energy of the kundalini usually returns to its latent state after some time, since most students cannot maintain this higher level of consciousness independently and consistently. Such an experience may transform and change the student's life, leading to increased creativity, energy and vitality and inspiring the student to work systematically to raise and channel that energy. In guiding such students, the teacher does not act on their own behalf but represents a tradition of spiritual gurus and masters, who direct the progress of those students who are prepared. Sloth and laziness are great obstacles on the path, for unless the student sincerely prepares, no teacher can help with the final steps.

TANTRA

Tantra yoga is the most misunderstood and abused of all practices. These sacred systematic and advanced practices for leading the aspirant to the highest state of consciousness have been caricatured in the West in a crude and superficial way. Tantra philosophy is the highest among all the practical philosophies of the East. In tantra yoga the chakras are used as centers of worship of Shakti, the primal force and mother of the universe. In tantra there are three schools: *Kaula, Mishra* and *Samaya*. These three schools are well established schools of philosophy in the world. Those who are spiritual teachers who have trained in a legitimate tradition so they can guide millions of people, have to properly study all three schools.

KAULA: Those who follow the Kaula tradition are actually worshipers of Shakti. They come from a tradition that knows the technique of living in the world yet remaining above. They use *panchmakaras* — *madya* (wine), *mudra* (dry grain), *maithun* (sexual intercourse), *mamsa* (meat) and *matsya* (fish). The Kaula school teaches how to organise the emotions and mental life. The Kaula school believes in focusing the mind at muladhara chakra as is demonstrated in particular geometrical diagrams. By studying this science of the school of Kaula, you can only have siddhis and worldly wisdom.

There are two principles in life in the universe — male and female. These two principles unite according to a certain process in order to awaken the kundalini. Two human beings prepare themselves and then they become one to awaken the kundalini. That is the Kaula method of external worship. Actually, swadhishthana is the place of worship according to the Kaula group. That is why in *Saundarya Lahari, Wave of Bliss and Wave of Beauty,* Shankaracharya bypassed that chakra because he was a swami. The Kaula group worships in swadhishthana where she is prepared to be wedded before going to manipura chakra. Those who want to acquire worldly wisdom and riches worship Shakti in swadhishthana. They use many methods. They get married, they have girlfriends or boyfriends, they drink alcohol and they take meat and fish. That particular worship is still used in many parts of India. Only one who knows the subject would recognize it. Those who practise it will never talk about this secret philosophy to anybody. Those families in Kerala, South India, who practise the Kaula method, are rare.

MISHRA: There is another community in India among the Brahmins called Mishras. *Mishra* means "combined" — internal and external worship. The Mishra group combines worldly success and devotion. Though they live in the world and are prosperous in the world they use devotion as a means to attain nearness. They want to know and see Devatma shakti, very closely, face to face! Actually, their forefathers were great tantrics and worshippers of Lord Shiva.

The Mishra group worships at anahata chakra, the heart center. This worship has the purpose of awakening the sleeping serpent-like fire without which a human individual soul remains primitive. They have different scriptures, but the scriptures do not provide much guidance because this is a very ancient tradition. Though the Vedas are considered to be the most ancient books, this tradition is equally as ancient as the Vedas. However, the instructions are given orally, for fear if they were written they would be lost or misused. When Buddha renounced the world and was enlightened, he went to Rajgiri and he charmed the whole world. Though many young people joined Buddha they did not know how to follow the discipline of renunciation so they created another *marga* (path), which is called *Vijnana*. Though taken from the scriptures, they misused the scriptures that were a part of Buddhism and destroyed the entire Buddhism. That's why there are no Buddhists in India. At the home of Buddha there is nothing. Outside India, Buddhism is flourishing.

In their way of worship they use 16 things, including manas puja, which sharpens the mind. If you attend your puja with sincerity and regularity, it makes your mind inward and one-pointed. They say mental worship is far superior to physical or external worship, the worship that is done by priests in the external world. Mind needs purification and needs to be prepared because mind can be a great obstacle. They say the fruits of any of your actions in the external world will remain in this world. Nothing goes with you, not your wealth, home, partner or children. Only your samskaras, the impressions that you have stored in the unconscious, will go with you. This is why you should immediately make effort to purify your mind.

SAMAYA: There is another marg that is called *Samaya* (I am with you). When you have this feeling that the divine mother is with you, and you are with her, then you follow this path. The school of Samaya is the highest path. It includes pure yogic exercises, mainly the science of breath and meditation. There are very few people who practise this path, because it is meant only for yogis. This school still exists in the Malabar Hills of South India. Those who understand this science are rare, though others talk much about it and write nonsense that misguides. Many western writers do not know what it is because we don't impart this knowledge to everybody. We test the students again and again and only then do we impart this knowledge. The center of worship in Samaya is ajna chakra. After you have done this worship, you have organized your emotional body and it no longer disturbs the lake of the mind, you are ready for the next step.

I was trained in the Samaya path in which you do not need to perform those rites that are meant for householders. The place of worship is the crown of the head, sahasrara chakra. To worship there you have to pass through a tunnel that is called *Brahmaguha,* and then by piercing the pearl of wisdom you go to *Brahmarandhra.* At the end of the tunnel there are three *bindus* (pearls) that are red, blue and white. That is why you will find colors that are symbols. For example, Shiva's color is blue, some of the gods look white and some of them look red. There are actually three bindus or gates that a sadhaka has to pierce before they can worship in sahasrara. There you will find Shiva and Shakti as one, although they may appear as two to you because of hypnosis. If you come out of hypnosis, you will see only one reality everywhere, within and without. As long as you are hypnotized, you will see many.

Maya is responsible for this manyness. *Ma* means "no," *ya* means "that." *Thou art not that.* It actually does not exist, but it seems to exist. One of the phases of maya is a *mirage.* For example, while going through a desert you may see a watery substance in front of you but the more you go toward the mirage the further away it seems to travel. You think that you live in the world and the world is real. However, this world is not real because it changes and does not stay as it is forever. That which changes cannot be called real. This so-called world is full of names and forms that change. If the form is changed, the name also changes. If you have some wood, you don't call it a table. If a carpenter makes that wood into a table, now you call it *table* because its form has changed. There is only one point for calling something real. Its origin has to be real; it has to come from truth. TRUTH MEANS THAT WHICH EXISTS FOREVER WITHOUT ANY CHANGE, DEATH OR DECAY.

The world is unreal because it is like a dream. In a dream you may be dreaming you have become a king and you are ruling the whole world, and even all of heaven is at your service. During your dream it was true that you were a king; that is dreaming reality. As dreaming reality is true for the extent of the dream, for a few years waking reality is also true. But like a dream it does not last for a long time. Therefore, this world is unreal. To live in the unreal world, you have to have a science. It is called lower knowledge or avidya, the knowledge that was imparted by the ancients. This includes how to perform your duties and how to do your practices in the world. Though they may be limited to sense gratification, they can lead you to heaven. And once your karmas are exhausted, you come down again although you are not liberated. You remain in bondage until you have destroyed all the fetters. Now, some people say, why do you want to destroy the fetters? Let us be born again and again with that consciousness of Brahman.

SAMADHI

SUTRA 3: *Tad evarthamatra nirbhasam svarupasunyam iva samadhih.*

THE PATH TO SAMADHI

According to yoga science, the purpose of meditation is to attain samadhi (enlightenment). Samadhi is the highest state in which you expand your consciousness to unite with the universal consciousness. Here, the seeker goes through *dharma megha samadhi,* beyond the normal laws of life to the unconscious. Some say you can go through the unconscious mind; others say you can go to the unconscious and be conscious there where you can let go of everything. And still others say you can bypass the unconscious. Once you have gone through the unconscious, then you will know yourself well. Otherwise, you know your body but you do not know anything about your breath or the various aspects of your mind or your soul. The secret is to have access to the unconscious mind any time you want without any hindrance.

You need more than human effort to experience samadhi. You have to prepare yourself to go beyond mind so you can come in touch with kripa (grace), the descending force. Suppose you do something so that your mind forgets all languages, all feelings of pain and pleasure and all thoughts of the past and imagining the future, what will happen to your mind? This is explained in *Kathopanishad.* When your senses are not distracted and your mind is tranquil, during that time you may attain a state of samadhi in which all your questions will be resolved. If you forget the languages in which your mind jabbers all the time and you know the method, you can attain that state of joy *(samahitam).* However, first you will have to cleanse the gross aspects of your mind of all ancient impurities. Enlightenment requires a free mind. That is why you have to practise japa, meditation, prayers and other methods to keep your mind focused on attaining that state of tranquillity where all your questions are resolved. Currently, you continue to put questions to your mind; mind replies by putting another question because it is never satisfied. When there are no more questions, mind will no longer be a source of disturbance and you will be in a state of tranquillity. That state of tranquillity cannot be maintained as long as there are questions. A day will come when all the thoughts accumulated in your unconscious mind will be exhausted and your mind will be free to attain samadhi, the highest rung on the yoga ladder where all problems and all questions are answered and solved. This state can easily be experienced in this lifetime if your meditation is one-pointed.

If you really want to enlighten yourself, you should learn to meditate systematically. From the very beginning there will be immense benefits. Meditation will help you to know yourself on all levels. The power of internal concentration will help lead you to the higher state of meditation. Dhyana (meditation) is the seventh rung of Ashtanga Yoga. A deep state of meditation should lead you to a state of tranquillity that prepares you to attain samadhi. And when you have enjoyed that state of tranquillity of which you are not ordinarily aware, that is the fourth state of turiya, or samadhi. Through the practice of these stages, one gradually advances to the higher reaches of consciousness, until one finally attains the state of samadhi—a state of pure consciousness in which one's individual soul becomes identified with the cosmic soul. That union is samadhi, the highest state of wisdom in which the individual soul unites with cosmic consciousness, like a drop uniting itself with the ocean. The deeper you dive into the ocean within, the more pearls you will be able to extract from the bottom of the ocean.

You perceive things according to the depth of your concentration and the capacity of mind. Thus, an ordinary mind and intellect will give you ordinary experiences, but the experience of samadhi is entirely different. To attain enlightenment does not mean to receive or achieve something. For a yogi, samadhi is considered to be the highest experience, because in that state mind does not function the way it normally does in ordinary day to day life. In samadhi, mind is completely purified, calm, inward and one-pointed. Such a mind will no longer disturb you. Freedom from bondage, ignorance and misery is the state of enlightenment, a state of perfection. When spiritual people experience samadhi, they will have similar, profound experiences, no matter from which tradition they come. WE ALL WALK IN THE SAME LIGHT so we will have similar experiences. Experiences come from various levels—sense experience, mental experience, spiritual experience and the ultimate experience of Brahman. In the state of samadhi one does not lose one's identity. In fact, as Patanjali has pointed out, it is only in the state of samadhi that you realize your true identity. This is not a negative state of being but a positive state of pure bliss and consciousness.

You think the highest of all joys is sleep. But unless you go beyond sleep to attain the state of turiya you cannot really see anything. Sleep is very close to samadhi. Samadhi means "oneness with the reality." Someone in deep sleep and someone in deep meditation are very close. That is why deep meditation is called sleepless sleep. If a fool goes to sleep they come out as a fool in the morning. Sleep gives rest, but sleep does not transform you or make you wise. But if you go into samadhi you will come out as a sage. One who says they are enlightened is egotistical;

one who doesn't say it is a fool. Only an enlightened person can recognize another enlightened person.

You are not yet aware that the highest of all joys is samadhi, where you remain fully aware and yet you are in deep sleep. This is why you have to learn the method of yoga nidra or conscious sleep. Ordinary sleep does not provide complete rest to the mind. In yoga nidra, even though you are in a deep sleep, you can record everything that is occurring around you. The whole world may believe that you are in a state of deep sleep, but actually you are fully aware and rested. In this way, you are giving your body complete rest, you are making your breath calm and your mind serene. One who knows the method of deep yoga nidra is very close to samadhi. One is a conscious act, the other is unconscious. You can attain that state simply by doing your duties skillfully in your daily life.

YOGA NIDRA

The finest time to practise yoga nidra is early in the morning before the sun rises, or in the evening around sunset. You should practise at the same time every day. The best time is right after meditation. It should be done when it is dark and there is no distraction or noise from outside, because even a little bit of noise can agitate your nervous system. This practice should not be used for sleep or for relaxation. If you see that you are falling asleep, try to break that.

1. Lie down in savasana. Do ten diaphragmatic breaths, exhaling and inhaling slowly and deeply. Or do a systematic relaxation.

2. Practise the 61 points exercise.

THE 61 POINTS EXERCISE

This exercise is also known as *shavayatra,* which means inner pilgrimage through the body. In this exercise awareness is directed and focused on 61 sacred points of the body. This exercise allows the student to closely inspect the body to discover where problems might lie, and also lead to a state of deep relaxation. Following the description of the exercise is a diagram that shows the location of these 61 points in the body.

Lie in the corpse posture or shavasana, with a pillow supporting your head.

Become aware of your breathing. Breathe deeply, smoothly and evenly, without any pauses or noise.

Then begin to release tension from the whole body, starting with the top of your head. Let go of tension in your scalp and facial muscles, neck and shoulders. From the shoulders, feel that release extend into the upper arms, elbows, lower arms, wrists, hands, fingers and finger tips.

Now, shift your attention to your chest, navel, lower abdomen and hips and release all tension from these areas. Then, from the hips allow the release to extend into the thighs, calves, ankles, feet and toes.

Then, reverse the direction of the release moving from your toes upward through the ankles, knees and hip joints.

Release tension from the whole pelvis, moving to your navel, chest, shoulders and neck. Then again release all tension from the face and scalp.

Continue to breathe deeply, smoothly and evenly without pauses or noise. Observe the quietness of the body as a whole.

Now, pay attention sequentially to the 61 special points of the body.

Bring your attention to the space between the eyebrows. Keeping your attention at this point, think of the number "1." Then, moving sequentially through the body, focus on the indicated number at each point.

Then, bring your awareness to the center of your throat, 2.
Right shoulder joint, 3.
Right elbow joint, 4.
Right wrist joint, 5.
Tip of the right thumb, 6.
Tip of the right index finger, 7.
Tip of the right middle finger, 8.
Tip of the right ring finger, 9.
Tip of the right little finger, 10.
Now come back up to the right wrist joint, 11.
Right elbow joint, 12.
Right shoulder joint, 13.
Bring your awareness to the center of your throat, 14.
Now go across to the left shoulder joint, 15.
Left elbow joint, 16.
Left wrist joint, 17.
Tip of the left thumb, 18.
Tip of the left index finger, 19.
Tip of the left middle finger, 20.
Tip of the left ring finger, 21.
Tip of the little finger of the left hand, 22.
Back up to the left wrist joint, 23.
Left elbow joint, 24.
Left shoulder joint, 25.
Bring your awareness to the center of the throat, 26.
Now bring your awareness down to the center between the two breasts, 27.

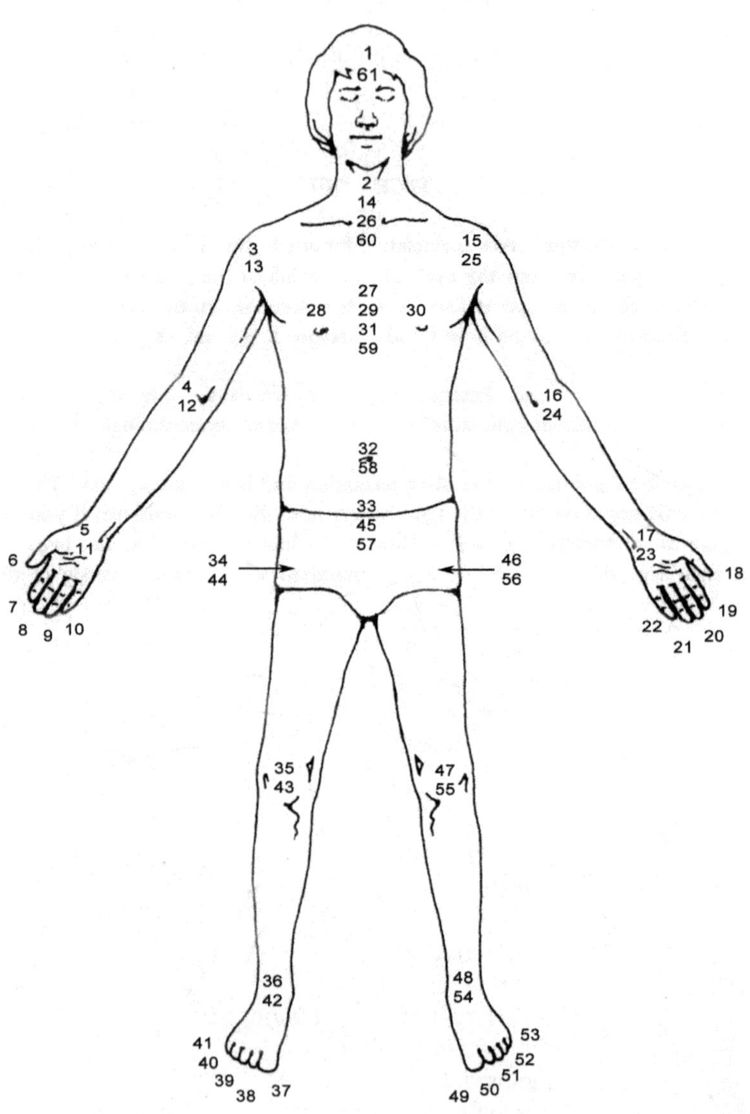

Then across to the right nipple, 28.
Back to the center between the two breasts, 29.
Across to the left nipple, 30.
Again back to the center between the two breasts, 31.
Now bring your awareness down to the navel center,
    32.
Come down to the pelvic center, 33.
Go across with your awareness to the right hip joint,
    34.
Down to the right knee joint, 35.
Right ankle joint, 36.
Now bring your awareness to the big toe of the right
    foot, 37.
Second toe, 38.
Middle toe, 39.
Fourth toe, 40.
Little toe of the right foot, 41.
Now come up to the right ankle joint, 42.
Right knee joint, 43.
Right hip joint, 44.
Back to the pelvic center, 45.
Now go across to the left hip joint, 46.
Left knee joint, 47.
Left ankle joint, 48.
Bring your awareness to the big toe of the left foot,
    49.
Second toe, 50.
Middle toe, 51.
Fourth toe, 52.
Little toe of the left foot, 53.
Come up to the left ankle joint, 54.
Left knee joint, 55.
Left hip joint, 56.
Come back to the pelvic center, 57.
Up to the navel center, 58.
Up further to the center of the chest, the heart center
    59.
Bring your awareness to the throat center, 60.
Come up to the center between the eyebrows, 61.

Continue to breathe deeply, smoothly, evenly and without a pause or noise for a few minutes. Feel as if you are breathing out and in through the eyebrow center.

This concludes the 61 point exercise.

After practicing this exercise for some time, you can visualize a blue or golden light at each of the 61 points instead of numbers.

OM, shanti, shanti, shanti.
OM, peace, peace, peace.

3. Then do shithali karana as follows:

SHITHALI KARANA

For the lower limbs repeat the exhalation and inhalation ten times. Then exhale and inhale five times from muladhara to sahasrara for each point above muladhara. When you inhale from the nostrils to the crown of the head your breath will become very short but deep and fine. During this time, your heart muscles and involuntary nervous system will rest, so your pulse and heart rate will decrease and your brain will also rest.

• Breathe ten times as if exhaling from the top of the head down to the toes and as if inhaling from the toes up to the top of the head.
• Exhale from the top of the head to the ankles and inhale from the ankles to the top of the head ten times.
• Exhale from the top of the head to the knees and inhale from the knees to the top of the head ten times.
• Exhale from the top of the head to the perineum at the base of the spine and inhale from the perineum to the top of the head five times.

• Exhale from the top of the head to the navel and inhale from the navel to the top of the head five times.
• Exhale from the top of the head to the heart center and inhale from the heart center to the top of the head five times.
• Exhale from the top of the head to the throat and inhale from the throat to the top of the head five times.
• Exhale from the top of the head to the bridge between the nostrils and inhale from the bridge between the nostrils to the top of the head five times.
• Exhale and inhale many times between the space between the eyebrows and the bridge between the nostrils.
• Exhale from the top of the head to the bridge between the nostrils and inhale from the bridge between the nostrils to the top of the head five times.
• Exhale from the top of the head to the throat and inhale from the throat to the top of the head five times.
• Exhale from the top of the head to the heart center and inhale from the heart center to the top of the head five times.
• Exhale from the top of the head to the navel and inhale from the navel to the top of the head five times.
• Exhale from the top of the head to the perineum at the base of the spine and inhale from the perineum to the top of the head five times.
• Exhale from the top of the head to the knees and inhale from the knees to the top of the head ten times.
• Exhale from the top of the head to the ankles and inhale from the ankles to the top of the head ten times.
• Breathe as if exhaling from the top of the head down to the toes and as if inhaling from the toes up to the top of the head ten times.

4. After doing each point with the proper number of breaths, turn onto your left side and breathe from head to toe and toe to head, breathing freely with

the whole right side of the body, without touching on any points. Breathe as though your whole right side is exhaling and inhaling ten times.

Then turn onto the right side and breathe as though your whole left side is inhaling and exhaling ten times.

Then shift onto your back and let your whole body inhale and exhale ten times, energizing your whole body with each inhalation and cleansing the whole body with each exhalation.

5. Now practise yoga nidra.

YOGA NIDRA

Let your mind come to ajna chakra, the space between the two eyebrows. Take three diaphragmatic breaths, letting go of your thoughts and even your mantra. Your eyes are closed and your breath is serene.

Next, with the help of your breath, shift your concentration to your throat. Visualize the moon at the throat chakra. Breathe freely without any conscious control, many times. Then breathe diaphragmatically.

Next, focus on the the heart center, anahata chakra. When you come to the heart center, make it the focal point and do diaphragmatic breathing.

Do not do the exercise for more than ten minutes. Your breath will become very fine. Go deep into the stillness and silence. Initially, remain in that deep stillness and silence for up to ten minutes, but no more. With practice, the length of time may increase, though this is not too important.

Then, systematically bring your attention outward from the stillness and silence, through the awareness of the relative quietness of the mind, the smoothness of the breath and the stillness of the physical body. Keep the deep stillness and silence with you as you gently move your fingers and toes. Then, open your eyes and slowly move as you wish.

LOVE WITHOUT AN OBJECT

You experience joy on different levels. *Joy* means "union." In the external world, to love an object or human beings gives you joy. You cannot imagine the joy you will experience when you unite with the center of consciousness. When you have tasted something very good, you cannot explain that taste to anyone else unless you share it with them. Similarly, the joy of samadhi is inexplicable. Mind, breath, senses and body are all externals and you are experiencing that great joy. But the HIGHEST OF ALL JOYS IS LOVE WITHOUT AN OBJECT. To realize that, you will have to learn to be quiet, calm and still in meditation.

SAMADHI AND SELF-TRANSFORMATION

SAMADHI IS LIKE ALCHEMY. It is a deep state of meditation that transforms a human being into a sage. When the student experiences the union of Shiva and Shakti at the sahasrara chakra, they experience samadhi, the highest state of consciousness in which they feel the presence of the Lord all the time. One who is constantly aware of the truth and yet living in the world free from the bondage of karma is enlightened. There are three stages. First, you become aware that YOU EXIST AND THE

LORD EXISTS. The next step is, I AM WITH THE LORD AND THE LORD IS WITH ME. And then, I AM THINE AND THOU ART MINE. But that is not the final stage. Jesus Christ said, *I and my father are one.* That is the last stage, the state of SELF-REALIZATION, which is UNION WITH THE UNIVERSAL CONSCIOUSNESS. You no longer have body, pranic, mental or ego consciousness, because your consciousness is the same as the consciousness of Brahman.

When you are enlightened you will become a perfect human being free from all misery, pain and suffering. Then you will no longer be lonely and you will be able to express your love. Sometimes you may think you have conquered your internal states. When you really have conquered your internal states, you will attain the highest state of samadhi, that state of perfect equilibrium and tranquillity that Patanjali describes. ENLIGHTENMENT DOES NOT CHANGE THE HUMAN BEING; IT TRANSFORMS THE PERSONALITY. Such a person knows themself and knows there is only one reality everywhere. That is freedom. If you can meditate for ten minutes continuously without any disturbance, I assure you, you will attain samadhi. But if you try to categorize your thinking process, you'll come to know even half a minute you could not meditate, though you sat for half an hour. I don't believe you when you say you do meditation for three hours. If you sit for three hours you will hallucinate. You cannot say hallucination is meditation. You can think for three hours, you can be aware of your thinking process for three hours, but if you can do three hours of uninterrupted meditation it means you are in samadhi.

SELF-REALIZATION

Many people say the highest of all worship is self-surrender, but the same scripture says Self-realization is the highest. There is a difference: here, the small self is the ego that should be surrendered. Self-realization needs awareness and experience. You say you are realized because you have realized you are a mortal being having a body and you are a breathing being with a conscious and unconscious mind. But this doesn't help to change your personality. Self-realization means realizing the self-existent truth that is already within you. Just as streams flowing into the ocean lose their names and forms, those who have realized the Self, having renounced their names and forms, lose themselves in the supreme Self that is higher than the highest.

Now, you may wonder how it is possible for anyone to be free. When a pot maker has made a pot they have performed their karma. The action of pot making gives them the fruit of the pots. But after they have made the pots, the wheel still revolves though it doesn't bear any fruits. Karma does not affect those who are enlightened, because they are like the wheel that has already produced the pots. They are rotating because they have to rotate. Even when one is enlightened, they can still desire to come back to the world to serve others. For such a person, there is no work to be done, because they are not in the bondage of death and birth. They live on the earth as free beings, helping and serving others and making people aware of the reality. They come to serve and to guide others. They come like lights or devas to this world, show the path and go away. This is one category of enlightened people.

Sometimes a spiritual desire can also cause problems. If you have the desire to attain, but you are not working with yourself you will remain restless and you will suffer because the flame is burning within you and you are not going according to your desire. If you have a spiritual desire to attain the highest reality and you do not direct your energies toward that, you may go through a series of depressions. You condemn yourself, you decide your life is of no use because you have wasted so many days, hours and years, yet you have not attained samadhi. Then, death will come and you will be reborn again. THE WORLD HAS NOTHING TO OFFER YOU AS FAR AS ENLIGHTENMENT IS CONCERNED, but if you learn to arrange the world around yourself, it will not create barriers and obstacles for you. If you continue to try to remove the obstacles, you will have no time to realize. Arrange your situation in such a way that there are no obstacles or barriers created in your family life, your social life and in your economical life. All the things that you have can be a means to freedom. Then, you will be free to meditate.

HOW LONG WILL IT TAKE

It naturally will take a long time to attain samadhi, but it certainly is possible for those who aspire for it and who persist to make efforts. It depends on how sincere you are and how much you have been practising. If you are not attached to anything of the world, you can be enlightened in a second's time. But that requires a radical change in your attitude and outlook toward the whole world, within and without. If you have a burning desire and firm determination you can enlighten yourself in a second's time. Enlightenment is not something you have to gain from outside yourself. If you really want to improve yourself in this lifetime, then you should decide from within to enlighten yourself. Even if a room is kept dark for hundreds of years, as soon as you light a lamp, the darkness is dispelled. Similarly, enlightenment is possible in one second's time. You have all the potentials: a body, a lifeline within the body and a light. If you BECOME AWARE OF THE LIGHT AND LIFE THAT ARE ALREADY WITHIN YOU, through which you think, see, hear, smell, taste, feel and move, then you will find that eternal source, and there can be no question of fear. This is the message of the ancient sages.

To reiterate, if you do not know the technique of withdrawal of the senses, you cannot have concentration, meditation or samadhi. Concentration becomes impossible if you do not learn how to pay attention toward the work that you have been doing. Meditation is not possible without concentration. And if you do not do meditation, samadhi is not possible. After a student has become firmly established in the preliminary practices of Ashtanga Yoga and has learned which posture will suit them best, has achieved some control and regulation of the breath and has withdrawn the mind from the objects of the senses, they are in a fit state to engage in the practices of concentration and meditation till they reach the stage of samadhi. When all activities of the mind are at a standstill and the mind is wholly absorbed in the Self, and there is no remaining shadow of anything else to distract its attention, the mind becomes like a flame that remains unshaken even by the breath of a breeze. This state of mind is a state of perfect peace, happiness and wisdom. It may last just a few seconds in the beginning, but its duration can be prolonged by practice and perseverance. When consciousness of the Self and its independence from all material objects becomes permanent and ever present to the mind, whether you are awake or asleep, you are emancipated. As one Upanishad declares, "The knots of the heart are sundered, all doubts disappear and all actions cease to exist once one has had a glimpse of Him."

SIDDHIS

"The SIDDHA IS a SPIRITUAL ALCHEMIST WHO
WORKS on and TRANSMUTES IMPURE MATTER, the
HUMAN BODYMIND, into PURE GOLD, the IMMORTAL
SPIRITUAL ESSENCE."
— GEORGE FEUERSTEIN

the POWER of MANTRA
SAMYAMA on SOUND
KNOWLEDGE of PAST BIRTHS
READING the MIND of ANOTHER PERSON
SAMYAMA on RUPA
NEGATIVITY
INVISIBILITY
SAMYAMA on FRIENDLINESS
SAMYAMA on STRENGTH
SAMYAMA on AHIMSA
SIXTH SENSE
SENSITIVITY
SAMYAMA on the HEART
PSYCHIC POWERS
SAMYAMA on the SUN
SAMYAMA on the MOON

THE POWER OF MANTRA

All the spiritual traditions of the world know how powerful the mantras are that have been imparted by the sages to their disciples. Once you have assimilated mantra, you can do amazing things. I have personally witnessed the tremendous power of mantra.

At Rishikesh there was a place called Jhari. *Jhari* means "bush." This was a place where swamis used to come and stay in small thatched cottages. One day they would come and the next day they would leave. This place was meant for those swamis who wander from one place to another rather than staying in any one place. It was very quiet there and nobody talked or disturbed the others that were staying there. One day I also went there with my master. He told me there was only one real swami among the 25 or 30 people that were staying there at that time. The old man he was referring to was a siddha (accomplished one). My master told me to go to him, observe him and learn from him.

Many disciples and masters used to come to learn from my master. Since I was very close to him from the very beginning I couldn't learn from him. Therefore, he would send me to other swamis to learn. As instructed by my master, I went to that old swami in the morning. We used to use a small twig from the neem tree for brushing our teeth. I watched as that swami went exactly to that branch of the neem tree where there was a very large hive of huge black killer bees. I shouted, "Swamiji, are you blind? Please gently retreat and come down!"

He was only two to three inches from that hive as he asked, "What is the problem?"

"The problem is those killer bees will kill you and they will also kill me!"

He said, "No. Killing comes from not understanding each other. This is why people are fighting all over the world. Nobody really wants to fight but they fight because they don't understand each other. I stay here and the bees know I am staying here. We have an understanding between us. I need to get a fresh brush from this neem tree every morning. So I climb, take one out and they don't do anything to me. I have told them, `You don't disturb me, and I won't disturb you.' They understand that. Animals understand better than human beings."

I was certain he was hiding some mantra from me so I asked him to share with me the mantra he was using. He agreed to give me the mantra. Before coming down, he told me to say, `I don't hurt you; you don't hurt me.'" Then, after taking a small twig from that tree, he came down and asked me to climb up, so I climbed up the tree. Because the swami was there, I was confident I could do as he said. He said, "Go very close to them and move. You will see nothing will happen."

"You want me to be killed?"

He said, "No one can kill you."

I said, "Will this mantra always help?"

He said, "It will always help."

So, I climbed the tree and just as he had told me, the bees didn't do anything to me. They would fly around me, but they did not disturb me, even though I was very close to them.

I was young and very much of a show-off during that time. So wherever I went to any village or city or anything, I would go outside the city and tell the people to find a tree where there was a hive, and I would show them a miracle.

There was a goldsmith at Bhavani. During those days it was in Punjab but now it is in Haryana. That goldsmith was very fat. He told me he knew where there was a hive. The swami who had given me the mantra had cautioned me that the mantra was only for me, not for others. Of course, I forgot that part. So I went to the tree and nothing happened. The bees did not misbehave. I said, "Now you go and say the same thing, 'I don't disturb you; you don't disturb me.'" All the bees immediately attacked him and he fell down! He remained in the hospital for eight days. His whole face and body were covered with bee stings. It was very difficult for the doctors to treat him.

No one can explain why this happened. Such mantras are called *apta* mantras. The qualities of apta mantras are different from those of other mantras. *Apta* means "someone gives you their own wealth out of pure love." Sometimes, with great delight the guru traditionally gives their student a mantra that is very powerful. That mantra usually works only for that student, but not for others. Yet, if he gives it with the same zeal to others, it also works. Apta mantras are like that. There may be one or several grammatical mistakes in apta mantras. Even so, we don't correct them but use them the way they are said. I have examined them many times.

I was a great coward for many years. Whenever I heard about a snake or saw a snake, my body would freeze. So my master gave me a mantra and told me, "Just remember this mantra and nothing will happen." And it worked for many years! Even when I used to walk in the forest where there were many wild animals such as tigers, bears, pythons, cobras and elephants, it would work. For many months I stayed on the other side of the Ganges without any shelter, sitting in the trees, living in caves and meeting many animals face to face, but no animal ever hurt me. I have seen its effect and I have seen others using it successfully.

Let me be alone means "don't make me lonely." Actually, if you're all alone, you're one with the reality and with the truth. But have you learned the way to really be all alone? For being all alone you'll have to be like a forest dweller and learn to be by yourself so you come to understand what solitude is. When you are all alone in the forest at night, you might have to walk where there are many wild animals. That is why in the cave they teach us to create a ring of light around ourselves. This can be done by bringing forward that pranic level of mind that is not only in the body but is also outside the body. Then no animal can come near you, or it would have a shock! Likewise, when you are in deep meditation, if somebody were to touch you with a finger, that person would also receive a shock. That is a sign of deep meditation and it can be recorded.

In 1939, when India was still under the rule of the British, a woman from Bengal was arrested at Lucknow railway station because she did not have a ticket. She asked the ticket taker how many tickets he wanted.

He said, "One."

She started to give him many proper tickets with the correct date.

Then he called the police and told them she had many stolen tickets. When the police arrived, she told them he was lying. "Ask him to give you those tickets." And he had nothing to give to the police.

Then, she went to the dining car and ate something. All of a sudden, coins started flying all over the car! And she said, "Pick up your money. These are the coins to pay for the food I have eaten."

Finally, when the train halted at Lucknow, the police arrested her. There is a cell at the railway station where they temporarily keep people who are under arrest. Then they try them in the court, and they are jailed according to the verdict. Even though the cell was locked, she could open it and would come out as she wanted. Six times they tried to lock her up with a huge lock, but still she was able to break it so she could come out. Then, she would stand outside and laugh. She enjoyed teasing all the people there. Nobody knew how to handle her. Finally, she said goodbye and got into the train that was going toward Nasik. Nobody knew what had happened to her after that.

Dr. Green and his party from the Menninger Foundation came to India to observe such phenomena and to make a movie. The night guard at the ashram asked why he had come. I told him he wants to see some unusual people.

The guard said, "I am one of them."

I did not think it was possible, but he proved me wrong. He put a sword in the fire; when the sword became red hot, he began to lick it. He was able to do that because he remembered a particular mantra. This is all in Dr. Green's movie.

You can also misuse mantras, and there are certain mantras that are used in black magic.

In 1938 there was a custom that in every police station there was one man who was called *bhavanti* inspector, who used to check and control black magic. I was staying in the house of a Mohammedan judge, because for me it was immaterial whether you were Christian, Hindu or Mohammedan. Because he kept misbehaving with his wife, she engaged someone who knew the science of black magic. So, anytime the judge would sign a check, that money would go to her. And many times he would vomit a bunch of needles. I saw it happen repeatedly.

This is called bhavanti vidya. When he found out who had helped that woman, he had that person arrested.

There are several hemispheres within the body. Three of these hemispheres are Rudrakhanda, Vishnukhanda and Brahmakhanda. Fire, water and kundalini come within Rudrakhanda. Then comes Vishnukhanda, which again includes fire, anahata chakra and vishuddha chakra. Next is Brahmakhanda. This journey is considered to be the highest of all. The teacher who wants a first class student to tread this path will lead them from here. On the other hand, the teacher will lead a second class student through many chakras. For a third class student it will take many lives.

When you are in meditation, you emanate power because you have attained the state of equilibrium where you are in touch with the center of love that is flowing equally for all. Tapas, the heat of meditation, is a very powerful thing. Only those who have been doing meditation will know what I am talking about.

Sant Jnaneshwar, one of the great sages of India, died at the age of 18 years. He was a very powerful man. When he talked about the fire and heat of meditation, the Brahmins did not believe what he was saying was true. So they said to him, "We are not going to listen to you because you are not Brahmin. You cannot even chant the Vedas."

He replied, "I will prove that I know the Vedas."

Then he called a buffalo to come to him and he told the buffalo to chant the Vedas. And so the buffalo started to chant the Vedas. He said, "You see, I am very powerful because I practise yoga. I am so powerful I can even make a buffalo chant the Vedas. Now what do you have to say, you Brahmins?"

And they said, "Okay, we believe you have power. Now, we want to see if you have another power. What is all this talk of meditational heat? We also do meditation."

He replied, "You do cold meditation."

Then he lay down and told them to put a pan or anything they wanted to heat on top of him. So they put a tawa on him and toasted many things on it. Finally, he said, "This is heat."

SAMYAMA ON SOUND

THE SOUND, THE IMAGE AND THE IDEA THAT ARE PRESENT TOGETHER IN THE MIND AT THE SAME TIME ARE IN A CONFUSED STATE. BY PERFORMING SAMYAMA ON SOUND, THAT CONFUSION IS RESOLVED AND THERE ARISES UNDERSTANDING OF THE MEANING OF ALL SOUNDS UTTERED BY ANY LIVING BEING.

You think sound is the very basis of communication, but that is not true. An idea and an image are behind the sound. Whenever you create a sound or you speak something, there is an idea, form and desire behind it. So, there are three things: the sound, the idea and the image that you have created. Before I came over here to speak to you, we had communicated. And after you go away, even then we will continue to communicate, because our communication does not depend on sound alone. No sound can come to you without form. A human being conceives the idea that creates a form. This whole world, this city and this building have all come from ideas. Beneath all the forms and images in your mind, there are ideas. It is the desire in the idea that creates a form. For example, somebody had a desire-filled idea and they built a house. So that idea is the actual builder of that house. When that idea mingles with the ideas of the family, the neighbors and the architect, then it becomes a house. So, many ideas must come together to make a house. Someone else came along and destroyed that house and then made it in a different way. This was also from an idea. Your thoughts have built your world, which is not the world manifested by the Lord, but the world you have created by yourself. Your problems do not come from the world that nature has manifested, but from the world you have created. Therefore, you should not project your problems onto others. You can very easily solve them if you try to understand them.

In your mind, there are many types of thought forms, symbols, ideas, fantasies and memories. If you study your thought forms you will find all thought forms are different from other thought forms. When you study the mental train of thought patterns you will come to know there are varieties of forms and every form has an idea behind it, and every idea has a desire behind it. Your actions are actually your thoughts, your thoughts are based on your emotions and your emotions are virtually your desires. When you desire something, that desire becomes the motivation that moves your whole being. So desire is the motivation for idea, idea creates the form and the form produces the sound.

KNOWLEDGE OF PAST BIRTHS

BY DIRECT PERCEPTION OF THE IMPRESSIONS THAT ARE RISING FROM THE UNCONSCIOUS YOU CAN GAIN KNOWLEDGE OF YOUR PREVIOUS BIRTHS.

Many of you are curious and very excited to know about your past. It's not difficult to find out what you were before. Initially, don't go to previous lives. Instead, you can easily find out what were you when you were five or six years of age. There is a big difference between what you were in your childhood and who are you today. I am not talking about regression. That is not the right way.

Yogis can know about their past births by systematically going to the bed of memories in the unconscious and by finally directly perceiving those impressions that are the source of motivation to come to this world. When you leave this world, you leave with certain unfulfilled desires. When you go to the unconscious and come in touch with those impressions that were the real motivation for you to come forward in this life, you can easily find out what you were in your past births. But why do you want to waste your time to know what you were before? If you come to know something about your past, how is it going to help you? This is why religious scriptures do not lead the student toward knowledge of past births. It would be better to use your time in what you want to become in the future.

When you go to sleep you go with certain unfulfilled desires. The next day, you wake up with those same desires and again you start to think about fulfilling those desires. You try to fulfill those desires in the daytime and again go to sleep. This has been going on for many centuries. When you die you still have certain desires to fulfill, and so you come back. Those desires again become motivation for you to return.

You will never be able to successfully do something for which you have not come, and you cannot continue to do something for a long time if you were not prepared to do that. Many people are not successful in what they are doing because they are not doing what they were meant to do. To educate a child, you should study the child's particular tendencies. Are they learning those habits from the external world, or are those habits based on past impressions and memories? Don't believe that anybody else is responsible for forcing you to come to this world or to go to another world; similarly, no one forces you to go to hell or to heaven. These are your own mental concepts. Each individual is fully responsible as they are the architect of this life and of their future life. One who studies and thus becomes aware of this will get freedom from the bondage of karma.

READING THE MIND OF ANOTHER PERSON

THROUGH SAMYAMA, YOU CAN DIRECTLY PERCEIVE THE IMAGE OCCUPYING THE MIND OF SOMEONE ELSE AND GAIN KNOWLEDGE OF WHAT THEY ARE THINKING.

You can penetrate into the thought forms of others even when they are not speaking to you. Then, if you study their thought forms and find out the desires behind them you can know what they are thinking. If you make your mind blank like a mirror for a few minutes, you will find images coming to you from the other person's mind. But when your mind itself remains preoccupied and creates many problems for you, your mind will not have the power to become a mirror that can reflect the other person's mind. This is very easy to do, but if you repeatedly do this, your mind will be completely distracted, and your efforts will be of no use. A mother unknowingly and unconsciously trains the child in the womb, just as the parents train the child in their childhood when the child is fast asleep. Wife and husband affect each other even during the sleep and dreaming states, just as two people sitting at the dining table in anger and not talking to each other can influence each other's emotional life. When you do not communicate with others, you hurt yourself and others too. Thought power is higher than the power of speech. In thought power there are three things mingled together: the image, the idea behind it and the desire behind the idea. Every image has a name and was built from an idea. That idea would never come if there were no desire. If you systematically study the form, idea and desire you can easily find out what others are thinking.

Once I met a man whose name was Mr. Touch. He was from the mountains of Almora in India. When he touched someone he could tell you everything about that person. But the moment he removed his finger, he could not say anything else. The Governor General of India at that time gave him the title of Mr. Touch. He went to the President's house and said he wanted to touch the Governor General. The guard told him he could not do that. He told the guard that unless he could touch him he could not use his power to help him. Slowly people came to know who he was and after some time he was given permission. He wanted to tell him there is a science of the mind, and by understanding that science one could improve. He did not eat anything before he went. And he said, "I have come to help him to improve because he is leading this country." This happened in the year 1946.

Mr. Touch was a very simple person, not very educated. When I asked him what the key to his success was he said he studies sensations. When I went to him, he did not know who I was, so I sat down and he touched me. But he said, "I am not receiving anything. What are you doing?" I realized that the way I practise to isolate myself from the atmosphere is the proper way and that it helps me.

He said, "Come out of that protective ring and then I will touch you."

I said, "If you cannot touch me in this condition, then I won't believe you."

He said, "No, I cannot work here."

I met another man at Rishikesh who used to charge 500 rupees for five minutes of his time. He was a Nepalese gentleman and he had cheated many people in Rishikesh in one day. It was his challenge that he would tell you only facts, but he wouldn't speak anything about the future. He said many things, none of which came true. That technique is called *karan vicharana*. He would listen to the sound vibrations coming from the right ear. When he was brought to me at my Ram Nagar ashram, I told people, "If he's really genuine, let him come over here and he will forget everything." I wouldn't have done that, but I thought this man was doing too much. It is not a good habit to rob people. Unfortunately, even learned swamis had started to follow him to learn this particular siddhi.

Among those who claim to study the mind, I have not met anyone who could study my mind, even though I went to them in a very humble and simple way. I even went to the most famous psychics. I said, "Tell me what is going on now in my mind and what has happened to me in the past, then I will believe what you say is going to happen to me in the future."

But these are insignificant things. Even if you know what I am thinking, this is not attainment. Attainment means to be able to direct my thinking on right lines. If you cannot transform my personality, that knowing will neither help you nor me.

One day when I was bathing on the bank of the Ganges I was thinking: *This old man troubles me so much. He has started to nag me and torture me constantly. This is not good. He has become such a problem. I think he should leave his body. Why did I tell him not to leave the body?* Such thoughts come in the mind and then pass. Once he said he wanted to leave the body. I told him if he were to leave his body, he would be a sinner. And I brought the scriptures where it was written if a teacher leaves his student ignorant he would go to perdition. Then he had assured me he would not leave his body at that time. Our cave was four miles away from that spot and I did not go to the cave for three days and there was no one with me. When I went to him I bowed as was my custom. He said, "Son, you seem to be fed up of me now." I denied it.

He said, "You never lie to me, but now you are lying. I was sitting next to you when you were thinking, *Oh, Lord, help me! He nags me so much.* Now I know you are fed up of me.

SAMYAMA ON RUPA

BY PERFORMING SAMYAMA ON RUPA, THE FORM, YOU WILL FIND OUT THE INITIATING IDEA, AND THE DESIRE OR MOTIVATION.

Do not go beyond the form. When you study the form from all angles then you can brood on the form and the thought images that are behind it. But do not study other mental factors that support the mental image for that is not the object of samyama. That which supports your mental object or any other object of mind is not considered to be samyama. Even if you know what somebody is thinking, don't think you have perfected samyama. You may have known the method of going to your internal states or the method of transformation of your three states. If you are able to make your mind one-pointed and inward, and you understand the form, image, idea and desire, this does not mean you have gone beyond the unconscious.

NEGATIVITY

Mind can also become negatively one-pointed. If you go on brooding on the same thing such as the conviction that you are going to die, you are surely going to die. And nobody can protect you. If you are constantly giving negative feedback to yourself or condemning yourself, there is no remedy in the world that can help you. Negative samyama is not good. Samyama should always be positively directed. Do not accept defeat either from adversity or from your own negative thinking—go on fighting with it. That is possible through will power.

INVISIBILITY

If I see you and your sense of sight is allowing you to see me, it means we are both receiving a sensation. The optic nerve carries that sensation to the brain and then to the conscious mind and unconscious mind. Now, if I see you I can learn to control that sensation I receive to such an extent that you will not be able to see me. If I don't allow you to perceive the form, you will not be able to see me. In such a situation, the yogi says you can make yourself become invisible. Many people think that to disappear is the same as becoming invisible. Actually, you are controlling the sensation of sight so that nobody can see you. There is no doubt at all in my mind that this is true. If you do samyama you can create that thought of a vision of someone so they do not exist for you. Then, you can walk into somebody's house and nobody will see you. Such experiments have been proven by many people, and they are not false.

SAMYAMA ON FRIENDLINESS

BY SAMYAMA ON FRIENDLINESS COMES THE STRENGTH OF THAT QUALITY.

Patanjali means any quality. If you are genuinely expressing friendliness, you will find strength in that. By performing samyama on friendliness, you can come to know how to be a friend to somebody. If someone thinks you are dishonest, you can never become their friend. To become someone's friend you have to learn three things: how to be faithful, sincere and truthful. If you find any of these three things lacking in yourself, then you cannot develop friendliness. If you understand what friendliness is, you cannot be a friend to someone and at the same time be dishonest. If you say you love somebody and sometimes you are dishonest to that person, that is not really love. You are just playing games. There are very few people who know how to truly love. We do not yet know what rules the center of emotions and feelings within. Some psychologists say that you cannot know unless you feel. Some say that you have to know first and then feel. Yet, knowing is a superficial level of mind and feeling is something deeper. Feeling is beyond reason, where reason cannot penetrate.

When you realize the strength that is already within you, that strength of gentleness that helps you to create friendship toward someone, then you come to know the laws that govern friendship between two individuals. Two true lovers are two entirely different things. Woman is neither inferior nor superior to man. It is difficult for man and woman to understand each other. Many times people compare and disturb their married life and friendliness, because they try to compare each other's behavior. But if you learn to love each other and understand the strength of love and friendliness, then you can understand the qualities that govern that friendliness. By meditating on those qualities you are constantly strengthening them. By becoming aware of those qualities and by expressing those qualities with mind, action and speech you can attain wisdom. First is friendliness, and then comes strength.

SAMYAMA ON STRENGTH

BY PERFORMING SAMYAMA ON STRENGTH, YOU CAN OBTAIN THE STRENGTH OF AN ELEPHANT.

The strength of friendliness is entirely different from the strength of animals. If a sage is very friendly, he does not have the strength of an animal. Likewise, if someone has the strength of an animal, it is not necessary that he also has the strength of friendliness. That is an entirely different level of strength. The law of association can be understood but if you devote your time to acquire the strength like the strength of elephant, you can do it.

If you are weak and you remain with sick people all the time, you will be affected by those sick persons. However, if you remain all the time with those who are strong, you will start to look after yourself and you will start to exercise to build your muscles. After sometime you will have attained something.

Once I met a swami who was making claims of having superhuman strength. That swami said, "Anybody can test me. And if you don't, I am going to test you."

One of the local rulers was driving a six-horse buggy. That swami caught hold of that buggy from behind so that the horses stopped abruptly. Even though the driver was using a whip to make the horses run, the horses were not moving. He got out of the buggy to see what the problem was. When he looked behind the buggy, he found it was the swami who was keeping it from going anywhere. He had terrific powers. This is an example of a human being's potential.

"Come on, make a bigger buggy, and I will again do it," declared the swami.

Don't think this is an old myth. I saw him do this and I also saw him catch hold of two buses with 50 persons aboard. He was able to stop those buses with powerful engines from going forward.

That swami died only a few years ago. There were others like Swami Ramananda, who could break elephant chains with his bare hands, but they were nothing before him. They all had learned bit by bit from him. His whole technique was control of prana and the energy sheath.

SAMYAMA ON AHIMSA

AHIMSA PRATISHTHAYAM TATSANNIDHO BIRATYAGA AHIMSA.

If you perform samyama on ahimsa (non-killing, non-harming, non-injuring, non-harming) on someone, even on a ferocious animal, they will become very loving and they will never hurt you.

SIXTH SENSE

BY DIRECTING THE LIGHT OF THE SUPER PHYSICAL FACULTY, KNOWLEDGE OF THE SMALL AND THE HIDDEN OR THE DISTANT IS OBTAINED.

In the external world, knowledge of the small can be gained by the microscope. You are inhaling millions of germs all the time, even though you cannot see them without a microscope. With a finer and more powerful microscope you can gain knowledge of the smallest objects that are not visible to the naked eye. Through a telescope you can see the sun, moon and stars. But without the help of any superficial thing, if you understand your super physical faculty, your sixth sense, you can know objects that are super small or extremely far away. This means anything that is hidden and is far away, that normally cannot be visualized by your eyes can be seen. There is something like a sixth sense that you cannot understand, but if you spend some time with someone who is blind, you will understand. There are many blind people who have been blind since birth. If you play cards with them and if you try to play any tricks on them, they will tell you not to be dishonest. They can do that because they have developed extreme sensitivity. When you learn to increase your sensitivity, that which is far away from you, beyond the reach of a telescope, your eyes and other instruments, you can know anything that is the smallest or which is hidden.

SENSITIVITY

The faculty of sensitivity is within you. Many times in your relationships in the world when you are not sensitive toward the pain, needs and desires of your partner, that becomes a source of difficulty that can finally lead to divorce. You all are sensitive as far as you are concerned with yourself, but you are not sensitive about the purpose of life or about the people whom you love because you are selfish. Selfishness leads you toward self-centeredness and contraction, and then you lose sensitivity. In love, you expand and give and grow; in contraction, you don't grow. Expansion is going toward consciousness; contraction is going toward selfishness.

By directing the life of the super physical faculty, knowledge of the small, the hidden, or the distant is attained. When you increase your sensitivity, you will not have to open your eyes to see something.

SAMYAMA ON THE HEART

You may think you have understood your mind because you understand certain theories of psychology and yoga. But it is not possible to know your mind without knowing your heart. The human mind and especially the human heart have tremendous powers. I am not talking about the physical heart; I am talking about anahata chakra, the heart that is not subject to the surgeon's knife. Anahata chakra is the subtle center situated between the two breasts that governs your body and the laws of life. If you are talking about the physical body, then manipura chakra or the solar system is the center. But now we are talking about the whole of life that includes mind, heart and body. Though many foolish people say the mind governs the heart, this is not true. IT IS THE HEART THAT GOVERNS THE MIND. The physical heart is definitely important, but more important is the spiritual heart that governs the physical heart and the mind. If you do not first understand the spiritual heart, your mind will not have much capacity. If you understand the laws that govern the spiritual heart, you can easily understand the nature of the mind.

According to Hindu mythology, when you go to a temple you will find four symbols that represent the four chambers of the heart. In the center lies Shiva on whom water is constantly dripping to create the sound *lub dub*. That external symbol makes you aware that in the heart within you is the center of meditation. By meditating on anahata chakra you will come to understand the mind and its nature. In Christianity it is called the Sacred Heart, while in Jewish literature it is the Star of David. And in Buddhist literature, this heart is the controller of your emotional life. At the time of initiation, the teacher recommends to those who are governed by their emotional life to concentrate on the spiritual heart. This will also help you to understand another person's thinking. Some people meditate on the spiritual heart for some time in order to gain knowledge of other persons' specifics such as their passport number and their father's and their children's names. They come to know just what is sufficient to make you think they must be a great sage. In this way they are able to earn a living. There are many people who do such things. But if you observe closely you will see they keep looking around for fear the police might come and arrest them. By doing samyama for some time, they acquire this skill and nothing beyond it. They are not concerned about the ultimate goal to realize the Self of all, the consciousness that is the fountainhead of all knowledge, peace and bliss.

PSYCHIC POWERS

You all are aware there is something like psychic power, and occasionally you may have had a hunch, though you have not been able to repeat it and you don't know how to be benefited by that. Now, scientists may not believe in psychic power. But many times it has happened that as I was remembering you, you have telephoned me. When two minds are in tune with each other, they can communicate mentally without speech or writing.

SAMYAMA ON THE SUN

BY PERFORMING SAMYAMA ON THE SUN YOU CAN GAIN KNOWLEDGE OF THE SOLAR SYSTEM AND UNDERSTAND THE LAW THAT GOVERNS ALL THOSE PHENOMENA.

Many fools misinterpret this sutra. They start to gaze on the sun and lose their eyesight after a few days. Samyama is not an external process, so gazing on the sun is not allowed. You are a universe yourself with an inner sun. Manipura chakra is your solar system, the biggest energy network in your system. The symbol of manipura chakra is a triangle that represents the upward-traveling flames of fire. If you know the governing laws of your solar system and learn to meditate on manipura chakra, the center of your solar system, then you will understand the organization of your whole body, because your body is governed by this solar system. If you understand how the internal solar system governs your body, you can easily acquire supernatural powers. Even if you do not know the governing laws, you can make use of certain powers, yet you will have no control.

There were yogis who knew the governing laws of the solar system and the science called SOLAR SCIENCE. For example, Jnaneshwara, Sant Eknath and several other sages, were able to perform miracles by meditating on the solar plexus. When Ramananda broke the elephant chain, his point of focus was his solar system. Paul Brunton was a great friend of mine when I was young. He was staying in India while he was writing the book *A Search in Secret India*. In that book he describes his experience with a swami he met at Banaras. He asked that swami if it were possible for somebody who is legally dead to be brought back to life. The swami replied that it could be done and that an animal or bird could be used to prove that it is possible.

So someone brought a dead bird to him that had been shot while it was flying. The bird had lain dead for several hours. The swami said that once the body goes through the process of decay, he would not be able to do anything. And he said to Paul Brunton, "If you want to know something about life and hereafter, observe what happens to this dead bird." And when it was declared dead, the swami put that bird between the two palms and whispered something. I wanted to know what he was whispering, but I could not catch it, because he was mumbling very quietly. Suddenly that bird took off and flew for quite a long distance. Paul asked the swami why he had not demonstrated this secret to the public and to the doctors. He said he would only share this knowledge with those who were selfless and do not have an ego problem, those who do not use healing to earn money.

Paul described another occasion, where he had witnessed a similar event in which the swami simply glanced at a bird and it fell down dead. He picked up the bird to confirm it was dead and that it was the same bird. In a few second's time the bird flew away and never returned.

Before they teach Kaula or Mishra, teachers first teach their students how to concentrate on the solar power at manipura chakra. The symbol of this chakra is situated at the navel in triangular form because the flames of fire go upward. After practising for a few days, they will begin to feel heat and start to perspire. In addition, their appetite will become excessive, so much so that they can eat 10, 20, even 40 plates of food in a day.

There was one saint, Neem Karoli Baba, about whom I have written in my book *Living With the Himalayan Masters.* Once when I was staying at his ashram he said to me, "These people are troubling my devotees, Bhole. Let's go." Bhole was my nickname. "I am going to teach them a lesson. They trouble us every day."

He then informed 40 of his disciples in the city that he was going to come and eat with them.

I said, "Why do you keep telling everybody that but you don't go anywhere? This is not good!"

He said, "No, this time you will come with me."

So I accompanied him. He asked me if I was happy, and I said yes.

Then he said, "I bless you."

He then began his epicurean adventure, going from one place to another until he had finished 40 plates that day. And he never stopped to go to the bathroom! Finally, when he sat down at the last place, he declared he was very hungry. This was because of the practice of concentration on manipura chakra.

I request those who are therapists and doctors to do some experiments on solar science. The more you meditate on manipura chakra the more your intuitive diagnosis ability will increase. I have proved it scientifically and it has been documented.

One day I was sitting in my office at the Menninger Foundation. One of the doctors came to inform me there would be a meeting at four o'clock. I asked him if it could be postponed until five because after taking food I sleep.

He said, "No. That's too late."

That day I did not eat much so I wouldn't feel too sleepy afterward. I went to that meeting even though I was half asleep while I was there. The doctor who had been treating the child whose case we were discussing knew I had been talking about intuitive diagnosis. She asked me what I thought was the child's diagnosis. The doctors involved with this case had said it was asthma.

I said, "No. In the third chamber there is a congenital hole and it needs to be treated."

One of the other doctors was considered to be an expert, and he became very angry. "Why are you challenging my knowledge?"

I replied, "I am not challenging anyone's knowledge. Take the patient to the lab and get it confirmed."

The tests confirmed there was a congenital hole in the heart.

Only therapists and doctors who have knowledge of anatomy and physiology can learn solar science and intuitive diagnosis. They should develop that ability through the practices of concentration on manipura chakra and agni sara to activate this chakra. When clinical symptoms or other findings fail, intuitive diagnosis can definitely help. It is unfortunate I was not able to train anybody in this country, because nobody wanted to do the preliminary work. It takes time, labor and effort.

SAMYAMA ON THE MOON

BY PERFORMING SAMYAMA ON THE MOON, ONE CAN GAIN KNOWLEDGE OF HOW THE STARS ARE ARRANGED.

If you understand the governing laws of the moon, you can understand the arrangement of the multitudes of stars. Patanjali says by meditating on the polar star, the knowledge of the movement of the other stars is acquired.

The average person's eyes are not sufficient to satisfy the whole power of the mind. My mind wants to see all the stars at one time, but my eyes are not capable of that.

Patanjali does not say you should practise to attain siddhis in order to attain the highest state of samadhi. These powers may help you to accomplish something in the world, but this should not be your goal. Some students stop their practices when they are confronted by stumbling blocks. They cannot go beyond because they do not want to lose the powers they have acquired. Others bypass the stumbling blocks and recognise these are obstacles in the path of Self-realization. Some yogis claim they are obstacles, while others say this is natural on the path of enlightenment. When you start to travel one after another to all the levels of your inner being, from subtle to subtler and then to the subtlest, you will automatically receive all these powers.

SILENCE
ALL WISDOM FLOWS from the SOURCE, the CENTER of SILENCE.

SILENCE DEFINED

INTUITION

OM

MEDITATION and SILENCE

KAIVALYA

SILENCE DEFINED

No one knows what silence means, but everyone aspires for peace and quiet. You would all like to be in deep silence at times, but you think you have to go somewhere to find silence. However, while you are away you keep thinking about the things you have left behind—your children, your home and your work. It is difficult for you to remain in silence because you are used to the rush and roar of modern civilization and you feel lonely when you are quiet. You have never tasted silence, even for a few minutes, because the mind becomes more active when you are quiet and is jabbering all the time. You should take some time for yourself and learn to be free with yourself, but when you get some quiet moments don't waste them by brooding on images from past impressions. One part of silence can be achieved by not allowing anybody to disturb you externally. A mother tells her children to please be quiet and to not disturb her. That quietness she is talking about is a desire, a longing for that height of silence where you don't have body, breath or sense consciousness. For that you will have to make effort.

Silence is not something external. For your mental health, it's important for you to understand quietness and stillness. Silence can give you something that no person or object can give you. When you sit down quietly, it does not mean your mind will immediately become quiet, because your thought forms do not stop. You have to calm down your chattering mind so you can enjoy that inner silence. A calm mind does not run here and there or produce fancies and fantasies. Even if you have learned to quiet your mind, another problem comes because the unconscious mind becomes more active. For silence, you need to direct your mind one-pointedly. When your mind is dissipated, you cannot know what silence is. You remain quiet when you close your eyes and you talk to your people with the images of your mind and you call this meditation. The day your mind consciously tastes silence, you will definitely enjoy that. And that enjoyment will continue to increase once you have experienced it. It will take a long time, but once you have understood and enjoyed the silence, you could easily get it again in a second's time without much effort. When a human being conducts their duties yet remains undisturbed in a state of balance that is quietness.

INTUITION

There is definitely something beyond this phenomenal world, which we term as divine. Human beings are composed of three qualities: *tamas, rajas* and *sattwa* (animal, human and divine). Usually, you conceptualize and come to certain conclusions based on sense perception, the knowledge you receive through your senses. This helps you to express yourself in the external world. However, when you dive deep into the recesses of human potential, you come to know that you have tremendous power. That power is intuition or divine potential. The finest knowledge you come in touch with is not in your body, breath or mind. It is beyond the mire of delusion created by your mind; it is in the silence within. The best of knowledge trickles from that silence where mind is calm, body is still and breath is serene. When you keep your head, neck and trunk in a straight line, body remains still. When you have done this, you will find that you are coming in touch with that wealth of knowledge which you were not aware of previously. You don't have to go to a teacher, lecturer, writer, swami or yogi to ask for confirmation of what you have experienced. Just like you never go to anybody to ask if you exist, because you know and know that you know. But that knowledge dawns from beyond all the fields of consciousness, external consciousness, all the superficial fields of consciousness and all the various aspects of mind.

In the final state of meditation, contemplation or prayer, you are not conscious of your body, senses, thought processes or emotions. This is the state of PERFECT SILENCE. During that time you might touch the infinite. And once you have touched infinity, you'll be free from all fears.

OM

The toughest and tersest Upanishad is *Mandukya Upanishad.* The whole gist of this Upanishad is contained in OM. OM is the first cosmic sound, the first syllable that was heard by Brahma. OM is the bow; atman, the individual self, is the arrow and Brahma, the universal Self, is the target. You have become an individual atman because you have a mind. In the first verse of *Mandukya,* mind is mentioned, but the rishis interpreted this as not the mere instrument of mind, but the whole unit of the individual soul.

OM is the eternal sound. If you hum any sound of any language with the lips closed, it will come out as OM. THE ENTIRE UNIVERSE IS CONTAINED IN THE SYLLABLE OM. In the Bible it is said in the beginning was the word and the word was God. Everything in the past, present and future is verily OM. Another name for the sacred sound OM is *pranava.* According to Patanjali, if you establish a bridge from this shore to the other shore with the help of pranava, you have accomplished your task. Pranava is a representative of the highest One that you are trying to attain. Some experts say pranava alone should not be used by worldly persons or by householders; it should only be used by sannyasas, those who have burned their desires in the fire of knowledge. Patanjali says you can use it to attain samadhi: *Tasya vacakah pranavah.* (sutra I.27) THE MANTRA PRANAVA IS THE REPRESENTATIVE OF THE CENTER OF CONSCIOUSNESS AND LEADS YOU TO THE CENTER OF CONSCIOUSNESS. When you go to see the president, a representative comes to greet you and leads you to the president. Mantra is like that representative. If you faithfully and sincerely follow it, it will lead you to the perfect silence. In deep samadhi you attain the undisrupted and unqualified highest state of silence.

Patanjali here brings the gist of *Mandukya Upanishad.* The entire philosophy and practice of the Upanishads has been summed into one. So is the case with mantra. Those who persist and remember their mantra can definitely attain the highest state. It's a spiritual wedding in which mantra weds the mind and leads the mind to silence. Nobody would want to wed a mind that is dissipated and scattered. But there is another silent state that is called turiya from where you can see all three states: sleeping, waking and dreaming.

There are mantras that create jerks in the breath and that is not healthy. The way to remember a short mantra is entirely different. If you do not know how to remember a short mantra such as OM you can hurt yourself. If you remember it very fast, *OM, OM, OM, OM, OM,* in your mind, your breath will slowly become shallow. Inhale while mentally prolonging the sound, *OMMMMMMMMMMMM,* and then exhale, *OMMMMMMMMMMMM,* with no pause in the breath. Remember the sound and meditate on the sound. This is the only sound that can be stretched without any problem or any jerks. Because mind is remembering a long mantra, the breath is extended also. Otherwise, the breath would become shallow.

According to Laya Yoga the first element earth is annihilated and it becomes water. Then, that becomes fire, and since fire evaporates anything liquid, water changes into air. Air transforms to space that is dissolved into sound. And finally, there is only one sound, OM. It was heard as OM by the great sages and they say it is OM. In Christianity they say it is *Amen.* They are one and the same. There is no sound better than OM because it represents the relationship between your soul and the Lord of life. Remember, all emotions are associated with your relationships. This emotion is related to your finest Self.

Previously, I have described how sound creates a pattern. If you say that a certain pattern will lead you to God, this is not true. First, you have to understand the meaning of the pattern. Another way to write OM in English is as A-U-M to represent the three states: waking, dreaming and sleeping. These are the three cities, but Tripurasundari actually dwells in the fourth, turiya (sleepless sleep). *Pura* means "city," *tri* means "three." All that you can do, your conscious functioning during the waking state is also her city, because of her power. The power you use during the dreaming state is also her power. And the power that leads you to sleep and gives you complete rest is also her power. But actually, her real state is turiya, sleepless sleep. THE SILENT OM IS TURIYA AND IS NOT SPOKEN.

If your mind is concentrated and it spontaneously flows toward the object, it will become easy for you to attain the next step. The object could be a figure or a light; it could be a mantra only and no image or nothing beyond that. The soundless state of OM is beyond time, space and causation. This is easy to understand with the following simile. If you stand on the banks of the Ganges or any river to find out from where the sound of the river is coming, you will never find the origin of the sound if you follow the flow of the river. You will have to follow the river upward from where it has originated and then come down. Then, finally you'll come to the place where there is no sound at all, the silence. ALL SOUNDS COME FROM THE SILENCE.

MEDITATION AND SILENCE

Meditation leads you to a state of joy and happiness where there are no questions. If there are no questions, no answers will be needed. Unless you understand how to sit, how to breathe, how to have a coordinated mind and how to go beyond into the absolute silence, you will never understand the silence. Remember that sloth is one of the biggest obstacles on the path of meditation. Practice makes one perfect, but that practice should be systematic. Don't leave your home in the morning unless you have meditated for a few minutes. The moment you wake up, sit down in meditation. Form the habit of practising meditation during the morning and evening hours. Gradually and gently you can establish tranquillity and harmony. When meditation is over, don't forget your mantra. Wherever you go, whatever you do, while doing your duties, you should remember your mantra. A time will come when you will no longer have to make conscious effort to remember your mantra. If you constantly remember your mantra, it will lead you to the meditative silence where the great Lord dwells. This is the source of the Ten Commandments that were given to Moses, the source of all the wisdom that came to Jesus, the source of all the wisdom of the Gita that came to Krishna and the source of the Light of Asia that came to Buddha.

Your target is to meet the beloved Lord of life. If you aim precisely with your arrow you will merge with the target and you will no longer need any arrow. Here, the word *precisely* is very important. If you do not practise shooting your arrows, they can go anywhere. It is the same in meditation. In the beginning, naturally the mind will run here, there and everywhere; but if you systematically do meditation, mind will not run anywhere. Mind runs when it has nothing on which to focus. You need to keep the mind focused so that mind is directed according to your intent. Mind always needs something to think of, some form. However, don't identify with the objects of your mind and don't allow mind to be a barrier. If you are always aware of Brahman you can go beyond to your essential nature that is peace, happiness and wisdom. To Krishna, all of Upanishadic literature was like a cow. He milked that cow and gave that milk to Arjun. That is how Arjun became great. *Arjun karna,* means "one who makes sincere effort." Here the student can make the bow from Upanishadic knowledge that has been acquired from the teacher. The aspirant should then fix the arrow of the mind one-pointedly to attain the goal of samadhi.

Set aside a time and place where you can be calm, still and in deep silence. We all are children of the silence and will go back to the silence. In the beginning was the word, the word was God, and God was the word. That beginning was silent. There were no distractions for body, breath, senses or mind. There you dwelled in your majesty and splendor.

You can exercise your gross muscles and control the voluntary nervous system, but you don't have control over your involuntary system. For that you need to learn to be still and to breathe in a serene way. It is very therapeutic and will bring you in touch with that dimension of life of which you are not yet aware. THE BEST OF KNOWLEDGE COMES THROUGH SILENCE. If you haven't known silence, then you haven't known anything.

While you are sitting to meditate you are constantly talking to your thought forms. This is not silence. Meditation helps you to go to the silence. May God lead you to the ultimate silence from where truth will be revealed to you. Ultimately, you will have to go to the silence within, the silence from where this whole universe has come, the fountain of peace, happiness and wisdom. EVERYTHING HAS COME OUT OF SILENCE. All this whatsoever you see here, there and everywhere is merely a projection of the ultimate silence. We are all products of silence. You want me to speak words of wisdom. Instead, you should want to share silence. Silence will give you ultimate peace, happiness and wisdom. FROM SILENCE AND QUIETNESS COME LIFE AND LOVE.

There was a great swami and students went to him. One of them asked, "Sir, please tell us about God."

He remained quiet.

The student persisted, "Sir, we have come from Delhi. You live in a Himalayan cave. We are simply requesting you to tell us about God. We can pay you."

Still the swami was quiet. After some time he finally spoke.

"I have been answering you, but you are not listening to me."

Puzzled, the student asked, "What do you mean?"

"GOD IS SILENCE."

There is nothing higher than the silence from which all peace, happiness and wisdom flow. With the help of meditation you can attain that silence and allow the reality to flow without any obstruction. All wisdom flows from the source, the center of silence. SILENCE ULTIMATELY GIVES PEACE, HAPPINESS AND WISDOM. This world has come from the silence and ultimately will return to the silence. Action and motion are only an intermediate state of the reality. All this whatsoever you see here, there and everywhere is merely a projection of the ultimate silence. THE FINAL REALITY is SILENCE.

KAIVALYA

Kaivalya is attained when there is equality of purity between the purusha and sattwa. KAIVALYA IS ABSOLUTE FREEDOM.

Index

Swami Rama

Swami Rama was born in the Himalayas and was initiated by his master into many yogic practices. His master also sent him to other yogis and adepts of the Himalayas to gain new perspectives and insights into the ancient teachings. At the young age of 24 he was installed as Shankaracharya of Karvirpitham in South India. Swamiji relinquished this position to pursue intense sadhana in the caves of the Himalayas. Having successfully completed this sadhana, he was directed by his master to go to Japan and to the West in order to illustrate the scientific basis of the ancient yogic practices. At the Menninger Foundation in Topeka, Kansas, Swamiji convincingly demonstrated the capacity of the mind to control so-called involuntary physiological processes such as the heart rate, body temperature and brain waves. Swamiji's work in the United States continued for 23 years, and during this period he established the Himalayan International Institute.

Swamiji became well known in the United States as a yogi, teacher, philosopher, poet, humanist, and philanthropist. His models of preventive medicine, holistic health, and stress management have permeated the mainstream of Western medicine. In 1993 Swamiji returned to India where he established the Himalayan

Institute Hospital Trust in the foothills of the Garhwal Himalayas. Swamiji left this physical plane in November, 1996, but the seeds he has sown continue to sprout, bloom, and bear fruit. His teachings, embodied in the words, "Love, Serve, Remember," continue to inspire the many students whose good fortune it has been to come into contact with such an accomplished, selfless and loving master.

Himalayan Institute
Hospital Trust

The Himalayan Institute Hospital Trust (HIHT) was conceived, designed, and orchestrated by Dr. Swami Rama, a yogi, scientist, researcher, writer, and humanitarian. The mission of HIHT is to develop integrated and cost-effective approaches to health care and development for the country as a whole, and for under-served populations worldwide.

Swamiji started this project in 1989 with an outpatient clinic of only two rooms. The hospital at HIHT currently has a thousand beds and is serving approximately 10 million people of Garhwal, Kumaon and adjoining areas. The hospital includes a Reference Laboratory, Emergency Wing, Operation Theaters, Blood Bank, Eye Bank, Dialysis Unit, I.C.U., C.C.U., Cath Lab., and a state-of-the-art Radiology Department. The Cancer Research Institute at HIHT is providing radiation therapy in addition to chemotherapy and surgical oncology.

The Rural Development Institute is providing health-care, education, income generation opportunities, water and sanitation programs, adolescent awareness programs and other quality of life improvement programs in the villages of Uttarakhand and adjoining rural areas.

The Himalayan Institute of Medical Sciences has become Swami Rama Himalayan University, a state university promoted by the Himalayan Institute Hospital Trust, and established by the Govt. of Uttarakhand under section 2(f) of UGC Act vide Act no. 12 of 2013. The University runs undergraduate (M.B.B.S.) and postgraduate courses (M.D./M.S. and Diploma) in 15 disciplines. The medical faculty also conducts paramedical degree courses in Medical Laboratory Technology, Radiology & Imaging Technology, and Physiotherapy. This University includes Himalayan College of Nursing, Himalayan School of Engineering and Technology, and Himalayan School of Management Studies.

The College of Nursing offers a 3-year GNM diploma program, a 4-year B.Sc. program, a 2-year Post Basic B.Sc. program and a 2-year M.Sc. program. The uniqueness of these nursing programs is that nursing students are provided hands-on training both in the community and with the rural population.

Two new departments have been added to the Faculty of Medicine: Dept. of Biosciences and the Dept. of Yoga Sciences and Holistic Health. The Dept. of Biosciences offers undergraduate and postgraduate degree programs in Biochemistry, Microbiology and Biotechnology. The Dept. of Yoga Sciences and Holistic Health currently offers a bachelor's degree program and plans to add a diploma program in the future.

In keeping with Swamiji's mission of integration, the hospital runs outpatient Ayurveda and Homeopathy clinics and the Ayurveda Center provides a residential pancha-karma therapy program for detoxification, rejuvenation and treatment of chronic ailments. The Combined Therapy Program, pioneered by Swami Rama, has been a unique model of holistic health care for more than 30 years. The Combined Therapy Program combines biofeedback, hatha yoga, aerobic exercise, nutrition, breathing, relaxation skills, meditation and other self-awareness techniques.

For information contact:

Himalayan Institute Hospital Trust
Swami Ram Nagar
P.O. Jolly Grant, Dehradun 248016
Uttarakhand, India
91-135-247-1200
pb@hihtindia.org
www.hihtindia.org

Swami Rama Society, Inc.

The Swami Rama Society is a registered, nonprofit, tax-exempt organization committed to Swami Rama's vision of bridging the gap between Western science and Eastern wisdom. The Society was established to provide financial assistance and technical support to institutions and individuals who are ready to implement this vision in the U.S.A. and abroad.

For information contact:
Swami Rama Society, Inc.
5000 W. Vliet St.
Milwaukee, WI 53208 U.S.A.
414-454-0500
info@swamiramasociety.org
www.swamiramasociety.org